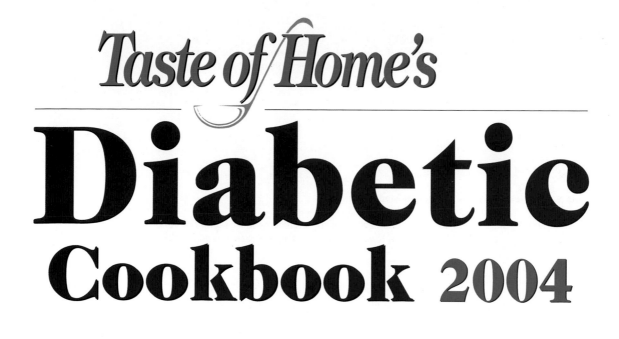

Taste of Home's
Diabetic
Cookbook 2004

Taste of Home Books

Recipe selection by Reiman Publications.

BISQUICK is a registered trademark of General Mills, Inc.

BREYERS® is a registered trademark owned and licensed by Unilever, N.V.

Fiber One® and Gold Medal® are registered trademarks of General Mills, Inc.

Some of the products listed in this publication may be in limited distribution.

Editor: Heidi Reuter Lloyd
Food Editor: Janaan Cunningham
Associate Food Editor: Diane Werner, R.D.
Recipe Editor: Janet Briggs

Nutritional Analysis: Linda R. Yoakam, M.S., R.D., L.D.

Front cover photography by Reiman Publications.
Food Stylist: Joylyn Jans
Food Photography: Rob Hagen, Dan Roberts
Senior Food Photography Artist: Stephanie Marchese
Food Photography Artist: Julie Ferron

Pictured on the front cover: Lime Cheesecake with Strawberries and Fresh Mint *(page 158)*.

Pictured on the back cover *(clockwise from top right):* Veggie Quesadilla Appetizer *(page 14)*, Pineapple Avocado Salad *(page 120)* and Mushroom Pasta Scampi *(page 96)*.

ISBN: 0-7853-9501-6

Library of Congress Control Number: 2003109987

Manufactured in China.

8 7 6 5 4 3 2 1

Nutritional Analysis: The nutritional information that appears with each recipe was submitted in part by the participating companies and associations. Every effort has been made to check the accuracy of these numbers. However, because numerous variables account for a wide range of values for certain foods, nutritive analyses in this book should be considered approximate.

Microwave Cooking: Microwave ovens vary in wattage. Use the cooking times as guidelines and check for doneness before adding more time.

Preparation/Cooking Times: Preparation times are based on the approximate amount of time required to assemble the recipe before cooking, baking, chilling or serving. These times include preparation steps such as measuring, chopping and mixing. The fact that some preparations and cooking can be done simultaneously is taken into account. Preparation of optional ingredients and serving suggestions is not included.

Taste of Home's
Diabetic Cookbook 2004

Personalizing Your Healthy Lifestyle

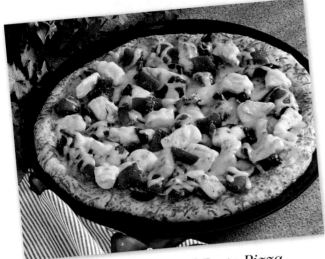

Marinated Chicken and Pesto Pizza (page 87)

EATING WELL JUST GOT EASIER

WELCOME to *Taste of Home's Diabetic Cookbook 2004,* the first edition of this new series. Before we go any further, let's put one common myth to rest.

You may think that people with diabetes need special foods prepared in special ways. Actually, the best recipes for someone with diabetes are no different than great recipes for everyone.

To prove that point, we've put together this cookbook. It offers an abundance of easy, delicious recipes your entire family will enjoy. As you look through the 224 recipes, you'll be surprised to see the wide variety of foods easily prepared with an assortment of delectable ingredients and seasonings.

These appealing recipes have been carefully created using low-fat, healthy ingredients that are readily available in most grocery stores. We cover the full range—from breakfast to dinner, plus desserts and snacks.

We've made this book easy to use with quick-glance symbols denoting low-fat, low-sodium, low-carbohydrate, high-fiber and meatless recipes. That way you don't necessarily have to look through the nutritional information to find a recipe that meets your needs. (See page 9 for a guide to the symbols used in this book and other helpful information.)

Preparation and cooking times are streamlined too, complementing today's busy lifestyles. In fact, the quick-to-make recipes are highlighted so you can easily find them without reading the entire recipe.

Unlike other diabetic cookbooks, these recipes bring family favorites to the table so your whole family can gain the rewards of eating well and enjoying every meal.

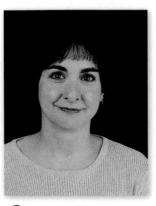

Diane Werner, R.D.

LOWERING FAT, NOT FLAVOR

Here are a few tips for increasing flavor without adding fat and calories:

Use herbs and spices liberally. Experiment with herb and spice combinations. Rub them onto meats before grilling, or sprinkle them over steamed veggies.

Instead of sautéing vegetables and meat in oil or butter, cook them in a little fat-free chicken or vegetable broth.

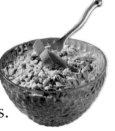

Reduced-fat and fat-free cottage cheese and cream cheese are great for making dairy-based dips and spreads.

Egg whites have the same leavening and binding properties as whole eggs, but without the fat from the yolk. Use them in a variety of dishes, such as quiches, casseroles, custards, cheesecakes, muffins and cookies.

To lighten up deep-fried appetizers such as egg rolls, use wonton skins and ravioli wrappers to enclose the savory fillings. Then bake them, instead of deep-fat frying.

Sweet red and yellow bell peppers and fresh garlic create great flavor without fat. Roast them, then use them to add texture and depth to soups, stews and sauces.

High-quality reduced-fat and fat-free cream cheese, sour cream and cheese are excellent substitutes for their full-fat counterparts. If you don't like the taste of one brand, try another.

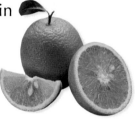

Citrus juices are well known for their tenderizing properties and the spark their tartness brings to dishes. Grated citrus peel (the skin without the underlying bitter white pith) gives an additional flavor boost. A little goes a long way.

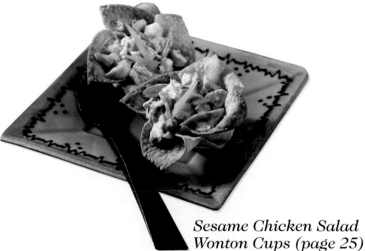

Sesame Chicken Salad Wonton Cups (page 25)

Personalizing Your Healthy Lifestyle **5**

MEAL PLANNING APPROACHES—EXCHANGES/CARBOHYDRATE COUNTING

People with diabetes can choose from several meal-planning approaches. Regardless of the plan used, one principle remains a common factor—all meal plans are designed to encourage you to eat similar amounts of carbohydrates at similar times each day.

EXCHANGE LISTS AND THE EXCHANGE SYSTEM

The exchange system categorizes foods into three main groups: carbohydrates, proteins and fats. An exchange system meal plan doesn't dictate what foods you eat. Instead, you choose from "exchange lists," lists of foods with similar nutritional make-up. For example, foods from the carbohydrate/starch group—such as a slice of bread, a small baked potato or 3/4 cup of unsweetened dry cereal—all have about the same amount of carbohydrate, protein and fat. Therefore, they are all exchangeable with each other.

An advantage of the exchange system is that it's still the common language used for communicating about food and diabetes. Cookbooks, magazine food articles, and even some food labels use it.

CARBOHYDRATE COUNTING

Carbohydrate counting is keeping track of the number of carbohydrate grams you eat each day, not the individual foods. An individualized meal plan is designed so you eat a specific number of carbohydrate grams at each meal and snack. You then choose foods that total the specified number of carbohydrates.

Carbohydrate counting is based on the fact that within one to two hours of eating, 90% to 100% of digestible starches and sugars turn up in your blood as glucose. So the amount of carbohydrate you eat may also determine the amount of medication you need to cover the rise in blood glucose from meals and snacks.

How do you know how many grams of carbohydrates are in foods? The Nutrition Facts panel on packaged foods lists the grams of carbohydrates in a serving.

Every recipe in this book lists grams of carbohydrates per serving, as well as the exchanges. An advantage of carbohydrate counting is you only keep track of carbs, instead of all components of your diet.

Q & A

1. Is honey better than sugar?
Honey is a source of concentrated carbohydrates and raises blood glucose as much and as quickly as other forms of sugar. Plus, it offers no nutritional advantages over other sources of sugar.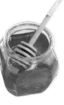

2. Your nutritional analyses do not list grams of sugar. Why not?
All carbohydrates, not just table sugar, cause a similar rise in blood glucose. It doesn't matter whether the carb comes from a potato or a candy bar; the body will treat it the same way. It's important for you to count all the carbs in your diet, and not focus just on sugar.

3. I'm a little confused about low-calorie sweeteners. Do they need to be counted in my meal plan?
Low-calorie sweeteners are "free foods." They make food taste sweet, yet have no calories and do not raise blood glucose levels. They do not count as a carb or any other exchange and can be

added to your meal plan instead of substituted.

4. What about these trendy diets? Would a low-carbohydrate diet be good for a person with diabetes?
Because these diets exclude a major food group, carbohydrates, they don't help people adopt the lifelong healthy eating habits that are key to weight loss success. They also lack many of the important nutrients found in fruits and grains.

If you are a person with insulin-dependent diabetes, much of your insulin needs have been determined based on the balance of your carbohydrate intake. Work with your diabetes care team to identify a healthy weight goal. Your team can help determine your calorie needs balanced with medication and exercise. You can lose weight the same way everyone else does, by taking in fewer calories and expending more.

RESTAURANT EATING

Here are some tips for eating out:

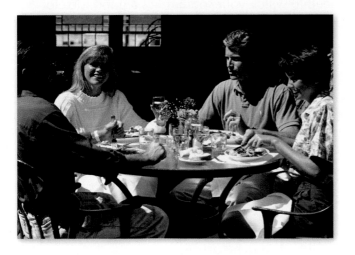

• If you're considering a restaurant you've never tried, stop by and look over the menu before you go in, to make sure you'll be able to order the meal you want. You won't be able to learn much about portion sizes, of course, but at least you'll know whether the menu includes acceptable options.

• If your meal is pasta heavy, order a side of steamed vegetables to mix in. The extra veggies add fiber and other nutrients. Save half for lunch the next day.

• Look for entrées that are grilled, steamed, baked without heavy sauces, broiled or prepared on a rotisserie.

• Ask for all dressings and condiments to be served alongside the meal so you can portion them out sparingly.

• Ask questions of the wait staff. For example, "How is the dish prepared? What are the ingredients? How large is the portion?" Then have it your way. If you like the burrito but don't want it smothered in sour cream, say so.

• Ask whether the kitchen can prepare half portions if regular portions seem too large, or ask that they box up half right away. Don't depend on your willpower to eat only half of what's in front of you.

• If you're really hungry when you go out, beware of the chips or rolls placed on the table before your meal. They contain a lot of empty carbohydrates that you must count in your meal plan. Instead, try ordering something more sensible to take the edge off your hunger—a side salad, a vegetable side dish or a glass of spicy tomato juice.

• If you must have butter for a roll or sour cream on a potato, ask for the lighter version. Most restaurants carry these but don't generally offer them as standard fare.

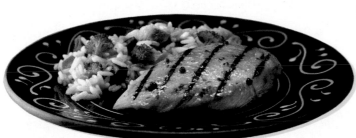

Grilled Chicken, Rice & Veggies
(page 75)

ABOUT PORTION SIZES

Food planning is of primary importance to a person with diabetes. When and how much you eat directly affects your blood glucose levels. If you are newly diagnosed, we encourage you to measure out portion sizes. This can help you learn what is considered a reasonable portion. After you have done this for awhile, you can then use these handy hand guides to help estimate portions.

Thumb tip = 1 teaspoon of mayonnaise, butter or salad dressing

Thumb = 1 ounce of cheese or meat

Tight fist = 1/2 cup of cooked pasta, starchy vegetables or unsweetened canned fruit

Handful = 1 cup (2 servings of pasta or 2 servings of cooked vegetables)

Palm = 3 ounces of cooked meat (no bone)

FOOD SELECTION TIPS

Here are a few ideas to help lighten up your shopping cart:

● Think lean, and choose cuts of meat with the words "round" or "loin." For example, ground round and pork tenderloin are leaner cuts.

● Reduced-fat dairy products are great nutritional investments that taste good. You can hardly tell the difference in a dip made with reduced-fat sour cream or a cheesecake made 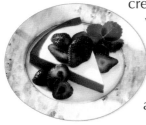 with light cream cheese. Save lots of fat and calories with reduced-fat cheeses sprinkled onto steamed veggies or even a veggie pizza.

● Experiment with reduced-fat margarines. They make a great spread for garlic toast and are equally great for making a lower fat graham cracker crust. You won't miss the butter!

● A variety of interesting canned beans are available. Beans aren't just for chili; they're excellent sources of fiber and lean protein. If you need to watch your sodium, it's a good idea to rinse them to get rid of some of the extra salt. Try adding them to soups and salads, or purée and season them for a healthy dip.

● Take advantage of supermarket offerings of pre-cut vegetables and packaged lettuces. Stock your freezer with frozen veggies. They'll be ready to add to your favorite dishes. Add them to soups, pasta dishes, you name it. Let your imagination go to work. Veggies are a great filler, and unless they're starchy, they can be great to fill up on, too.

● Learn more about herbs, spices, flavored vinegars and even oils. You will be surprised at the intense flavor they give to foods. For example, a simple mixture of freshly minced gingerroot, garlic and reduced-sodium soy sauce makes a wonderful fat-free marinade for grilled meat.

● Ready-to-eat, low-fat low-sugar cereals provide extra crunch and flavor when used as toppings on fruit, yogurt or baked vegetables.

● Increase your use of whole grains such as barley. One cup of cooked barley packs about 6 grams of fiber. This fat-free grain contains complex carbohydrates, B vitamins and protein. It makes a great addition to soups, casseroles, salads and chili.

● Try a no-calorie butter spray found in the dairy section of your grocery store. Use it on corn on the cob in place of butter or spray it on vegetables, chicken or fish fillets to help seasonings adhere to the food.

● Purchase some fat-free salad dressings and use them for more than just lettuce salads. They make good marinades and dressings for pasta salad and are even great drizzled over hot cooked veggies.

● Try evaporated fat-free milk in place of whole milk or cream in sauces, soups and baked goods.

HOW WE CALCULATE NUTRITIONAL ANALYSES

● When a choice of ingredients is given in a recipe (such as 1/3 cup of sour cream or plain yogurt), the first ingredient listed was the one used for calculating the Nutrients per Serving.

● Recipe or plate garnishes were not included in our calculations.

● Optional ingredients were not included in our calculations.

● When a range is given (such as 2 to 3 teaspoons), we calculated with the first amount listed.

● Only the amount of the marinade that is absorbed during preparation was calculated.

ABOUT THE ICONS

You will find special icons included with many recipes in the book. With these, you can determine at a glance which recipes fit your needs. Here is a simple explanation of the icons:

 low fat 3 grams or less per serving

 low sodium 140 milligrams or less per serving

 low carb 10 grams or less per serving

Quick Recipe: 30 minutes or less total preparation and cook time

 high fiber 5 grams or more per serving

meatless includes eggs and dairy products

cooking for 1 or 2 recipe serves 1 or 2 people

ADDITIONAL RESOURCES

If you have not met with a diabetes educator or attended a diabetes education class, ask your doctor or healthcare provider about educational opportunities. A registered dietitian can help you make good food choices and also help you understand your personal meal plan.

For general information about diabetes, visit the American Diabetes Association's Web site at **www.diabetes.org** or call 1-800-342-2383.

To locate a diabetes educator in your area, contact the American Association of Diabetes Educators at **www.aadenet.org.**

The American Dietetic Association can provide customized answers to your questions about nutrition. Visit their Web site at **www.eatright.org** or call 1-800-366-1655.

The *Diabetic Newsletter,* which is published every other Monday, can be sent directly to your e-mail address. The newsletter contains general information, recipes and frequently asked questions with answers. To subscribe, visit **http://diabeticnewsletter.com.**

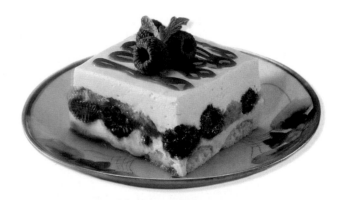

*Lemon Raspberry Tiramisu
(page 161)*

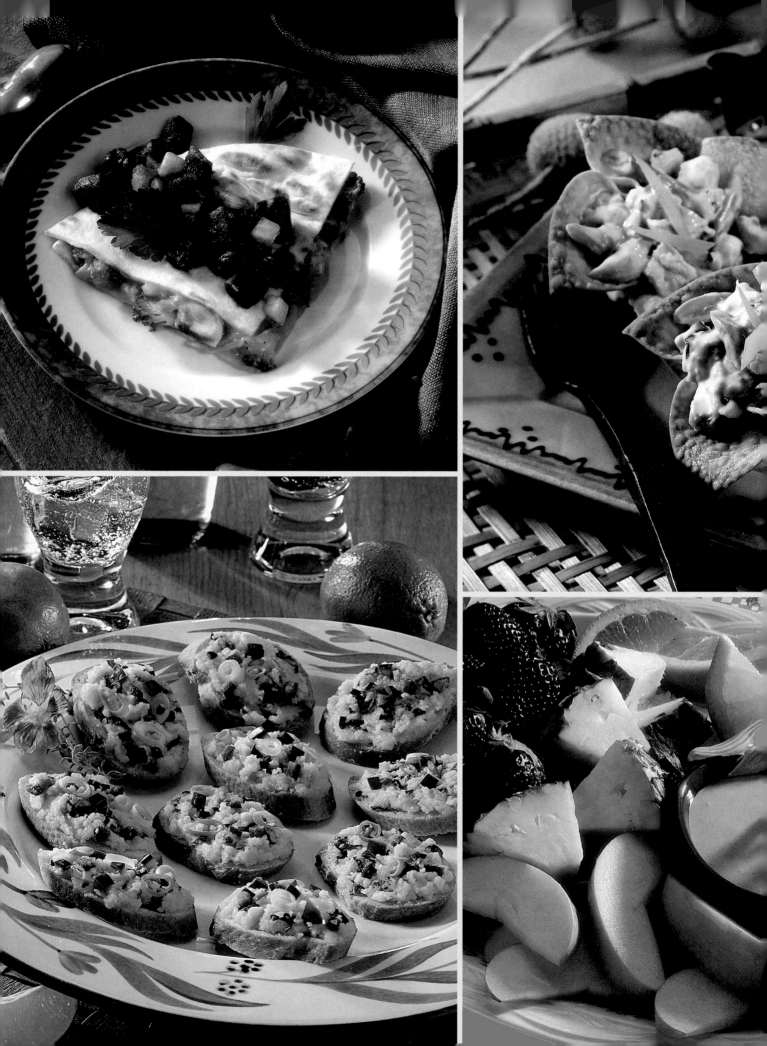

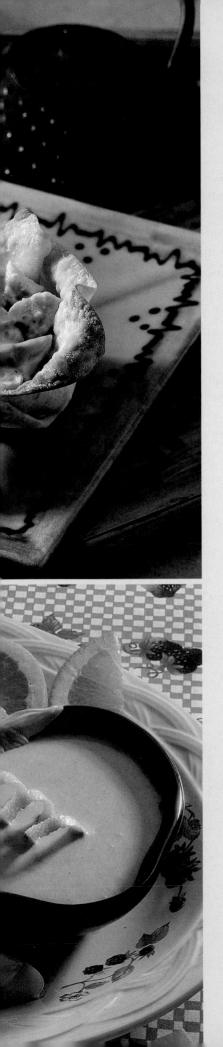

Appetizers

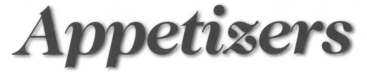

🍂 🍂 🍂

Berry Good Dip

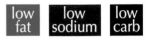

Quick Recipe   *(Pictured at left)*

8 ounces fresh or thawed frozen unsweetened strawberries
4 ounces fat-free cream cheese, softened
1/4 cup reduced-fat sour cream
1 tablespoon sugar

1. Place strawberries in food processor or blender container; process until smooth.

2. Beat cream cheese in small bowl until smooth. Stir in sour cream, strawberry purée and sugar; cover. Refrigerate until ready to serve.

3. Spoon dip into small serving bowl. Garnish with orange peel, if desired. Serve with assorted fresh fruit dippers or angel food cake cubes.   *Makes 6 (1/4-cup) servings*

Nutrients per Serving: 1/4 cup Dip (without fruit dippers and cake cubes)

Calories 47	**Fiber** 1g
Fat 1g (sat <1g)	**Cholesterol** 7mg
Protein 3g	**Sodium** 120mg
Carbohydrate 6g	

Exchanges: 1/2 fruit, 1/2 lean meat

Clockwise from top left: Veggie Quesadilla Appetizer (page 14), Sesame Chicken Salad Wonton Cups (page 25), Berry Good Dip, and Toasted Pesto Rounds (page 18)

Black Bean Quesadillas

Quick Recipe *(Pictured at right)*

> Nonstick cooking spray
> 4 flour tortillas (8 inches)
> 3/4 cup (3 ounces) shredded reduced-fat Monterey Jack or Cheddar cheese
> 1/2 cup canned black beans, rinsed and drained
> 2 green onions with tops, sliced
> 1/4 cup chopped fresh cilantro
> 1/2 teaspoon ground cumin
> 1/2 cup salsa
> 2 tablespoons plus 2 teaspoons fat-free sour cream
> Chopped fresh cilantro, for garnish (optional)

1. Preheat oven to 450°F. Spray large nonstick baking sheet with cooking spray. Place 2 tortillas on prepared baking sheet; sprinkle each with half the cheese.

2. Combine beans, green onions, cilantro and cumin in small bowl; mix lightly. Spoon bean mixture evenly over cheese; top with remaining 2 tortillas. Coat tops with cooking spray.

3. Bake 10 to 12 minutes or until cheese is melted and tortillas are lightly browned. Cut into quarters; top each tortilla wedge with 1 tablespoon salsa and 1 teaspoon sour cream. Transfer to serving plate. Garnish with chopped fresh cilantro, if desired. *Makes 8 servings*

Nutrients per Serving: 1 Quesadilla wedge (with 1 tablespoon salsa and 1 teaspoon sour cream)

Calories 105	**Fiber** 1g
Fat 4g (sat 1g)	**Cholesterol** 8mg
Protein 7g	**Sodium** 259mg
Carbohydrate 13g	

Exchanges: 1 starch, 1/2 lean meat

Marinated Artichoke Cheese Toasts

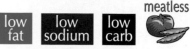

Quick Recipe

> 1 jar (8 ounces) marinated artichoke hearts, drained
> 1/2 cup (2 ounces) shredded reduced-fat Swiss cheese
> 1/3 cup finely chopped roasted red peppers
> 1/3 cup finely chopped celery
> 1 tablespoon plus 1-1/2 teaspoons reduced-fat mayonnaise
> 24 melba toast rounds
> Paprika

1. Rinse artichokes under cold running water; drain well. Pat dry with paper towels. Finely chop artichokes; place in medium bowl. Add cheese, peppers, celery and mayonnaise; mix well.

2. Spoon artichoke mixture evenly onto melba toast rounds; place on large nonstick baking sheet or broiler pan. Broil 6 inches from heat about 45 seconds or until cheese mixture is hot and bubbly. Sprinkle with paprika. Garnish, if desired. *Makes 12 servings*

Nutrients per Serving: 2 Toasts

Calories 57	**Fiber** 1g
Fat 1g (sat 1g)	**Cholesterol** 4mg
Protein 4g	**Sodium** 65mg
Carbohydrate 7g	

Exchanges: 1/2 starch

Tip

Look for roasted red peppers packed in cans or jars in the Italian food section of your supermarket.

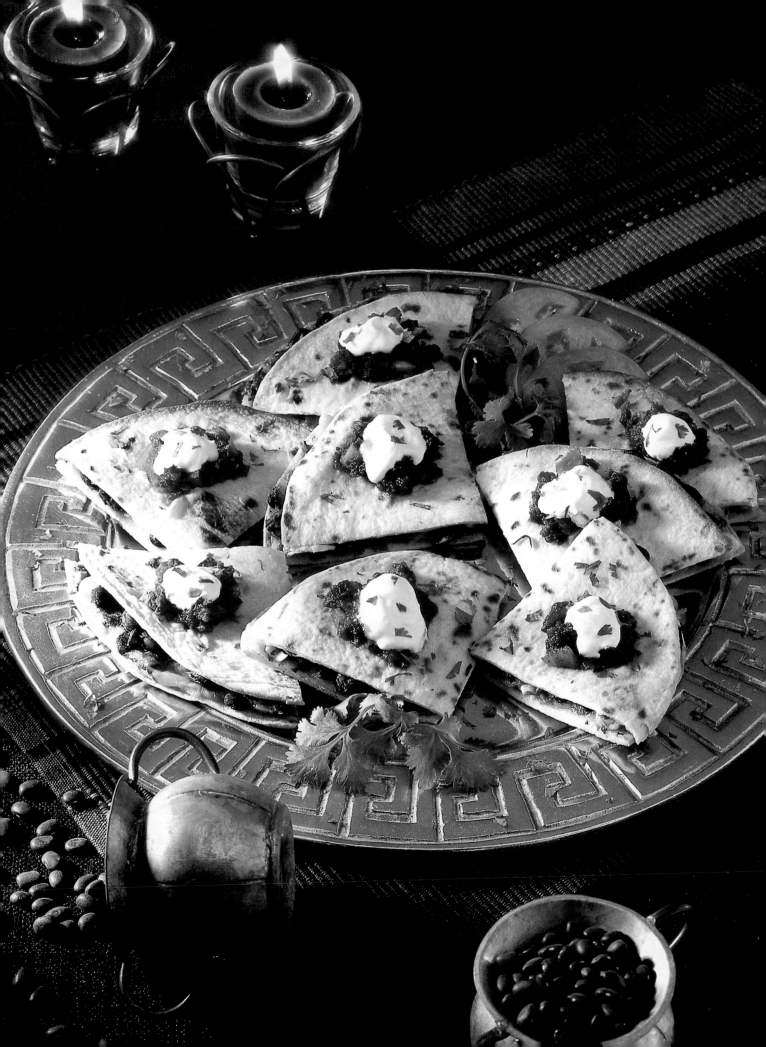

Veggie Quesadilla Appetizers

(Pictured on page 10)

10 flour tortillas (8 inches)
1 cup finely chopped broccoli
1 cup thinly sliced small mushrooms
3/4 cup shredded carrots
1/4 cup chopped green onions
1-1/4 cups (5 ounces) shredded reduced-fat
sharp Cheddar cheese
2 cups Zesty Pico de Gallo (recipe
follows)

1. Brush both sides of tortillas lightly with water. Heat small nonstick skillet over medium heat until hot. Heat tortillas, one at a time, 30 seconds on each side.

2. Divide vegetables evenly among 5 tortillas; sprinkle evenly with cheese. Top with remaining 5 tortillas.

3. Cook quesadillas, one at a time, in large nonstick skillet or on griddle over medium heat 2 minutes on each side or until surface is crisp and cheese is melted.

4. Cut each quesadilla into 4 wedges. Serve with Zesty Pico de Gallo.

Makes 20 servings

Zesty Pico de Gallo

2 cups chopped seeded tomatoes
1 cup chopped green onions
1 can (8 ounces) tomato sauce
1/2 cup minced fresh cilantro
1 to 2 tablespoons minced jalapeño
peppers*
1 tablespoon fresh lime juice

*Jalapeño peppers can sting and irritate the skin; wear rubber gloves when handling peppers and do not touch eyes. Wash hands after handling peppers.

Combine all ingredients in medium bowl. Cover and refrigerate at least 1 hour.

Makes 20 servings

Nutrients per Serving: 1 Quesadilla wedge with about 1-1/2 tablespoons Zesty Pico de Gallo

Calories 79	**Fiber** 1g
Fat 2g (sat 1g)	**Cholesterol** 4mg
Protein 4g	**Sodium** 223mg
Carbohydrate 12g	

Exchanges: 1 starch

Cheesy Spinach Dip

1 cup reduced-fat sour cream
1 cup low-fat (1%) cottage cheese
1 box (10 ounces) frozen chopped
spinach, thawed and squeezed dry
1 can (8 ounces) sliced water chestnuts,
drained and chopped
1 package (1.4 ounces) instant vegetable
soup mix
1/4 cup (1 ounce) grated Parmesan cheese
2 tablespoons milk (plus additional milk,
if necessary)
1-1/2 teaspoons dried chives
Cut-up raw vegetables and crackers
(optional)

1. Combine sour cream, cottage cheese, spinach, water chestnuts, instant soup mix, Parmesan cheese, milk and chives in large bowl; mix well. Cover and refrigerate at least 2 hours or overnight.

2. Stir well before serving. Add more milk if dip is too thick. Serve with raw vegetables and crackers, if desired.

Makes about 3-1/2 cups dip

Nutrients per Serving: 2 tablespoons Dip (without extra milk)

Calories 34	**Fiber** 1g
Fat 1g (sat 1g)	**Cholesterol** 4mg
Protein 3g	**Sodium** 187mg
Carbohydrate 3g	

Exchanges: 1 vegetable

Festive Franks

Quick Recipe (Pictured at right)

1 can (8 ounces) reduced-fat crescent roll dough
5-1/2 teaspoons barbecue sauce
1/3 cup finely shredded reduced-fat sharp Cheddar cheese
8 fat-free hot dogs
1/4 teaspoon poppy seeds (optional)
Additional barbecue sauce (optional)

1. Preheat oven to 350°F. Spray large baking sheet with nonstick cooking spray; set aside.

2. Unroll dough and separate into 8 triangles. Cut each triangle in half lengthwise to make 2 triangles. Lightly spread barbecue sauce over each triangle. Sprinkle evenly with cheese.

3. Cut each hot dog in half; trim off rounded ends. Place one hot dog piece at large end of one dough triangle. Roll up jelly-roll style from wide end. Place point-side down on prepared baking sheet. Sprinkle with poppy seeds, if desired. Repeat with remaining hot dog pieces and dough.

4. Bake 13 minutes or until dough is golden brown. Cool 1 to 2 minutes on baking sheet. Serve with additional barbecue sauce for dipping, if desired.   *Makes 16 servings*

Nutrients per Serving: 1 Festive Frank

Calories 77	**Fiber** 0g
Fat 3g (sat <1g)	**Cholesterol** 8mg
Protein 4g	**Sodium** 385mg
Carbohydrate 8g	

Exchanges: 1/2 starch, 1/2 lean meat, 1/2 fat

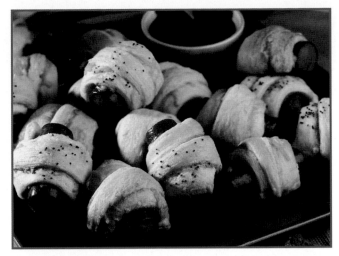

Festive Franks

Eggplant Caviar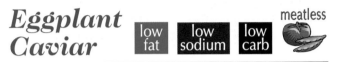

1 large eggplant, unpeeled
1/4 cup chopped onion
2 tablespoons lemon juice
1 tablespoon olive or vegetable oil
1 small clove garlic
1/2 teaspoon salt
1/2 teaspoon TABASCO® brand Pepper Sauce
Sieved hard-cooked egg white and lemon slices (optional)

Preheat oven to 350°F. Place eggplant in shallow baking dish. Bake 1 hour or until soft, turning once. Trim off ends; slice eggplant in half lengthwise. Place cut-side down in colander and let drain 10 minutes. Scoop out pulp; reserve pulp and peel. Combine eggplant peel, onion, lemon juice, oil, garlic, salt and TABASCO® Sauce in blender or food processor. Cover and process until peel is finely chopped. Add eggplant pulp. Cover and process just until chopped. Place in serving dish. Garnish with egg white and lemon slices, if desired. Serve with toast points.   *Makes 1-1/2 cups*

Nutrients per Serving: 1 tablespoon Eggplant Caviar (without toast points)

Calories 10	**Fiber** 1g
Fat 1g (sat <1g)	**Cholesterol** 0mg
Protein <1g	**Sodium** 45mg
Carbohydrate 2g	

Exchanges: Free

Citrus Cooler

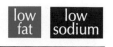

Quick Recipe   *(Pictured at right)*

- **2 cups fresh squeezed orange juice**
- **2 cups unsweetened pineapple juice**
- **1 teaspoon fresh lemon juice**
- **3/4 teaspoon vanilla extract**
- **3/4 teaspoon coconut extract**
- **2 cups cold sparkling water**

Combine juices and extracts in large pitcher; refrigerate until cold. Stir in sparkling water. Serve over ice.   *Makes 9 servings*

Nutrients per Serving: 2/3 cup Citrus Cooler

Calories 59	**Fiber** <1g
Fat <1g (sat <1g)	**Cholesterol** 0mg
Protein <1g	**Sodium** 1mg
Carbohydrate 13g	

Exchanges: 1 fruit

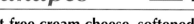

Crab Canapés

- **2/3 cup fat-free cream cheese, softened**
- **2 teaspoons lemon juice**
- **1 teaspoon hot pepper sauce**
- **1 package (8 ounces) imitation crabmeat or lobster, flaked**
- **1/3 cup chopped red bell pepper**
- **2 green onions with tops, sliced (about 1/4 cup)**
- **64 cucumber slices (about 2-1/2 medium cucumbers cut 3/8 inch thick) or melba toast rounds**
- **Fresh parsley, for garnish (optional)**

1. Combine cream cheese, lemon juice and hot pepper sauce in medium bowl; mix well. Stir in crabmeat, bell pepper and green onions; cover. Chill until ready to serve.

2. When ready to serve, spoon 1-1/2 teaspoons crab mixture onto each cucumber slice. Place on serving plate; garnish with parsley, if desired.   *Makes 16 servings*

Tip: To allow flavors to blend, chill crab mixture at least 1 hour before spreading onto cucumber slices.

Nutrients per Serving: 4 Crab Canapés made with cucumber slices

Calories 31	**Fiber** <1g
Fat <1g (sat <1g)	**Cholesterol** 5mg
Protein 4g	**Sodium** 178mg
Carbohydrate 4g	

Exchanges: 1/2 lean meat

Avocado Salsa

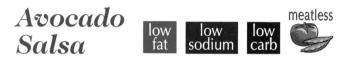

- **1 medium avocado, peeled and diced**
- **1 cup chopped seeded peeled cucumber**
- **1 cup chopped onion**
- **1 Anaheim or other mild chili,* seeded and chopped**
- **1/2 cup chopped fresh tomato**
- **2 tablespoons chopped fresh cilantro**
- **1/2 teaspoon salt**
- **1/4 teaspoon hot pepper sauce**

*Chili peppers can sting and irritate the skin; wear rubber gloves when handling peppers and do not touch eyes. Wash hands after handling peppers.

1. Combine avocado, cucumber, onion, chili, tomato, cilantro, salt and hot pepper sauce in medium bowl; mix well.

2. Refrigerate, covered, at least 1 hour to allow flavors to blend. Serve as a dip or condiment.   *Makes about 4 cups or 32 servings*

Nutrients per Serving: 2 tablespoons Avocado Salsa

Calories 13	**Fiber** <1g
Fat 1g (sat <1g)	**Cholesterol** 0mg
Protein <1g	**Sodium** 38mg
Carbohydrate 1g	

Exchanges: Free

Citrus Coolers

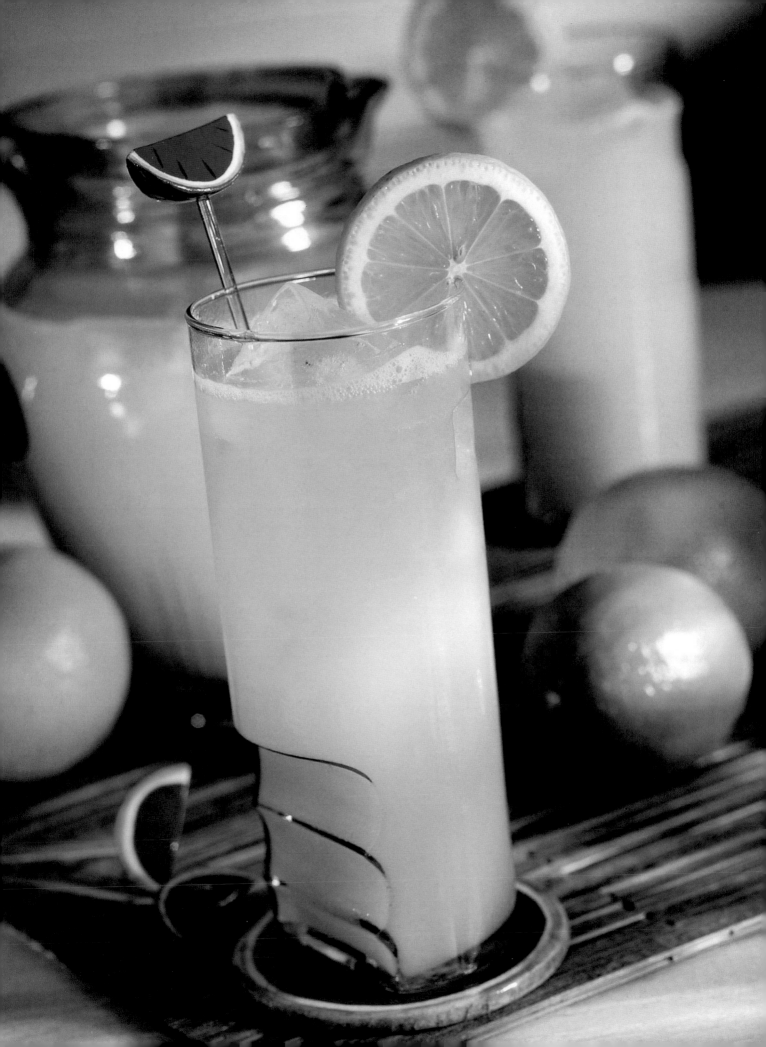

Toasted Pesto Rounds

Quick Recipe   *(Pictured on page 10)*

> 1/4 cup thinly sliced fresh basil or chopped fresh dill
> 1/4 cup grated Parmesan cheese
> 3 tablespoons reduced-fat mayonnaise
> 1 medium clove garlic, minced
> 12 French bread slices, about 1/4 inch thick
> 1 tablespoon plus 1 teaspoon chopped fresh tomato
> 1 green onion with top, sliced
> Black pepper

1. Preheat broiler.

2. Combine basil, cheese, mayonnaise and garlic in small bowl; mix well.

3. Arrange bread slices in single layer on large nonstick baking sheet or broiler pan. Broil 6 to 8 inches from heat 30 to 45 seconds or until bread slices are lightly toasted.

4. Turn bread slices over; spread evenly with basil mixture. Broil 1 minute or until lightly browned.

5. Top evenly with tomato and green onion. Season to taste with pepper. Transfer to serving plate.   *Makes 12 servings*

Nutrients per Serving: 1 Pesto Round

Calories 90	**Fiber** <1g
Fat 2g (sat 1g)	**Cholesterol** 3mg
Protein 3g	**Sodium** 195mg
Carbohydrate 14g	

Exchanges: 1 starch, 1/2 fat

Potato Pancake Appetizers

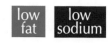

> 3 medium Colorado russet potatoes, peeled and grated
> 1 egg
> 2 tablespoons all-purpose flour
> 1 teaspoon salt
> 1/4 teaspoon black pepper
> 1-1/2 cups grated zucchini (2 small)
> 1 cup grated carrot (1 large)
> 1/2 cup reduced-fat sour cream or plain yogurt
> 2 tablespoons finely chopped fresh basil
> 1 tablespoon chopped chives *or* 1-1/2 teaspoons chili powder

Preheat oven to 425°F. Wrap potatoes in several layers of white paper towels; squeeze to remove excess moisture.

Beat egg, flour, salt and pepper in large bowl. Add potatoes, zucchini and carrot; mix well.

Coat 2 nonstick baking sheets with nonstick cooking spray. Place vegetable mixture by heaping spoonfuls onto baking sheets; flatten slightly.

Bake 8 to 15 minutes until bottoms are browned. Turn; bake 5 to 10 minutes more.

Stir together sour cream and herbs; serve with warm pancakes.

Makes about 24 appetizer pancakes

Favorite recipe from **Colorado Potato Administrative Committee**

Nutrients per Serving: 1 Pancake with 1 teaspoon herbed sour cream

Calories 30	**Fiber** 1g
Fat 1g (sat <1g)	**Cholesterol** 11mg
Protein 1g	**Sodium** 106mg
Carbohydrate 5g	

Exchanges: 1/2 starch

Rice & Artichoke Phyllo Triangles

low fat | low sodium

(Pictured below right)

1 box UNCLE BEN'S® Butter & Herb Fast Cook Recipe Long Grain & Wild Rice

1 jar (6-1/2 ounces) marinated quartered artichokes, drained and finely chopped

2 tablespoons grated Parmesan cheese

1 tablespoon minced onion or 1 green onion with top, finely chopped

1/3 cup plain nonfat yogurt or fat-free sour cream

10 sheets frozen phyllo dough, thawed

1. Prepare rice according to package directions. Cool completely. Preheat oven to 375°F. In medium bowl, combine rice, artichokes, Parmesan cheese and onion; mix well. Stir in yogurt until well blended.

2. Place one sheet of phyllo dough on a damp kitchen towel. (Keep remaining dough covered.) Lightly spray dough with nonstick cooking spray. Fold dough in half by bringing short sides of dough together; spray lightly with additional cooking spray.

3. Cut dough into four equal strips, each about 3-1/4 inches wide. For each appetizer, spoon about 1 tablespoon rice mixture onto dough about 1 inch from end of each strip. Fold 1 corner over filling to make triangle. Continue folding as you would fold a flag to form a triangle that encloses filling. Repeat with remaining dough and filling.

4. Place triangles on greased baking sheets. Spray triangles with nonstick cooking spray. Bake 12 to 15 minutes or until golden brown.

Makes 40 appetizers

Tip: Use a pizza cutter to cut the phyllo dough into strips.

Nutrients per Serving: 1 Triangle

Calories 34	**Fiber** <1g
Fat 1g (sat <1g)	**Cholesterol** 1mg
Protein 1g	**Sodium** 129mg
Carbohydrate 5g	

Exchanges: 1 vegetable

Today's Slim Line Dip

low fat | low carb

Quick Recipe

1 cup dry curd cottage cheese
1/2 cup buttermilk
1/4 teaspoon lemon juice
1 package dry onion soup mix

Add cottage cheese, buttermilk, lemon juice and onion soup mix to food processor or blender. Process until smooth. Refrigerate. Serve with raw vegetables.

Makes 16 servings (about 2 cups)

Favorite recipe from **Wisconsin Milk Marketing Board**

Nutrients per Serving: 2 tablespoons Dip (without vegetables)

Calories 40	**Fiber** 1g
Fat 1g (sat <1g)	**Cholesterol** 1mg
Protein 3g	**Sodium** 883mg
Carbohydrate 6g	

Exchanges: 1/2 starch

Rice & Artichoke Phyllo Triangles

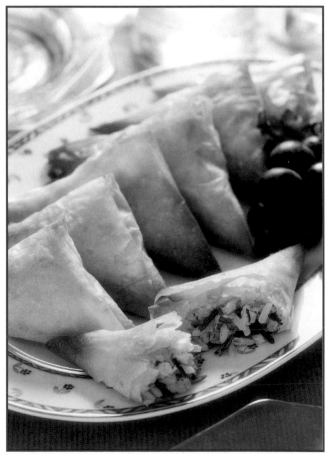

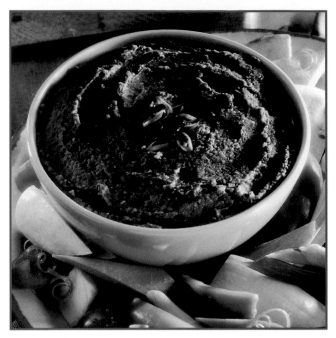

Garlic Bean Dip

Garlic Bean Dip

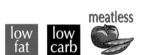

Quick Recipe   *(Pictured above)*

> **4 cloves garlic**
> **1 can (15-1/2 ounces) pinto or black beans, rinsed and drained**
> **1/4 cup pimiento-stuffed green olives**
> **1 tablespoon plus 1 teaspoon lemon juice**
> **1/2 teaspoon ground cumin**
> **Assorted fresh vegetables and crackers**

Place garlic in food processor; process until minced. Add beans, olives, lemon juice and cumin; process until well blended but not entirely smooth. Serve with vegetables and crackers. Garnish, if desired.

Makes 12 servings (about 1-1/2 cups)

Nutrients per Serving: 2 tablespoons Dip (without vegetables and crackers)

Calories 42	**Fiber** 1g
Fat 1g (sat <1g)	**Cholesterol** 0mg
Protein 3g	**Sodium** 207mg
Carbohydrate 7g	

Exchanges: 1/2 starch

Leek Strudels

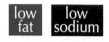

> **Nonstick cooking spray**
> **2 pounds leeks, cleaned and sliced (white parts only)**
> **1/4 teaspoon caraway seeds**
> **1/4 teaspoon salt**
> **1/8 teaspoon white pepper**
> **1/4 cup fat-free reduced-sodium chicken broth***
> **3 sheets thawed frozen phyllo dough**
> **Butter-flavored nonstick cooking spray**

*To defat chicken broth, skim fat from surface of broth with spoon. Or, place can of broth in refrigerator at least 2 hours ahead of time. Before using, remove fat that has hardened on surface of broth.

1. Coat large skillet with nonstick cooking spray; heat over medium heat. Add leeks; cook and stir about 5 minutes or until tender. Stir in caraway seeds, salt and pepper. Add chicken broth; bring to a boil over high heat. Reduce heat to low. Simmer, covered, about 5 minutes or until broth is absorbed. Let cool to room temperature.

2. Preheat oven to 400°F. Cut each sheet of phyllo lengthwise into thirds. Spray 1 piece phyllo dough with nonstick cooking spray; spoon 2 tablespoons leek mixture onto bottom of piece. Fold 1 corner over filling to make triangle. Continue folding, as you would fold a flag, to make triangular packet.

3. Repeat with remaining phyllo dough and leek mixture. Place packets on cookie sheet; lightly coat tops of packets with butter-flavored cooking spray. Bake about 20 minutes or until golden brown. Serve warm.

Makes 9 servings

Nutrients per Serving: 1 Leek Strudel

Calories 52	**Fiber** 1g
Fat 1g (sat <1g)	**Cholesterol** 0mg
Protein 1g	**Sodium** 107mg
Carbohydrate 11g	

Exchanges: 2 vegetable

Spicy Orange Chicken Kabob Appetizers

low fat **low sodium** **low carb**

2 boneless skinless chicken breasts (about 8 ounces)
1 small red or green bell pepper
24 small fresh button mushrooms
1/2 cup orange juice
2 tablespoons reduced-sodium soy sauce
1 tablespoon vegetable oil
1-1/2 teaspoons onion powder
1/2 teaspoon Chinese five-spice powder

1. Cut chicken and pepper each into 24 (3/4-inch) square pieces. Place chicken in large resealable plastic food storage bag and peppers and mushrooms in another resealable food storage bag.

2. Combine orange juice, soy sauce, oil, onion powder and five-spice powder in small bowl. Pour half over chicken and half over vegetables. Close bags securely; turn to coat. Marinate in refrigerator 4 to 24 hours, turning frequently.

3. Soak 24 small wooden skewers or toothpicks in water 20 minutes. Meanwhile, preheat broiler. Coat broiler pan with nonstick cooking spray.

4. Drain chicken and discard marinade. Drain pepper and mushrooms, reserving marinade. Thread 1 piece chicken, 1 piece pepper and 1 mushroom onto each skewer. Place on prepared pan. Brush with marinade; discard remaining marinade.

5. Broil 4 inches from heat source 5 to 6 minutes or until chicken is no longer pink in center. Serve immediately.

Makes 12 servings

Nutrients per Serving: 2 Kabobs

Calories 30	**Fiber** <1g
Fat <1g (sat <1g)	**Cholesterol** 10mg
Protein 4g	**Sodium** 38mg
Carbohydrate 2g	

Exchanges: 1/2 lean meat

Mexican Roll-Ups

low fat **low carb**

(Pictured below)

6 uncooked lasagna noodles
3/4 cup prepared guacamole
3/4 cup chunky salsa
3/4 cup (3 ounces) shredded fat-free Cheddar cheese
Additional salsa (optional)

1. Cook lasagna noodles according to package directions, omitting salt. Rinse with cool water; drain. Cool.

2. Spread 2 tablespoons guacamole onto each noodle; top with 2 tablespoons salsa and 2 tablespoons cheese.

3. Roll up noodles jelly-roll fashion. Cut each roll-up in half to form 2 equal-size roll-ups. Serve immediately with additional salsa, if desired, or cover with plastic wrap and refrigerate up to 3 hours.

Makes 12 appetizers

Nutrients per Serving: 1 Roll-Up

Calories 40	**Fiber** 1g
Fat 1g (sat 0g)	**Cholesterol** 2mg
Protein 3g	**Sodium** 218mg
Carbohydrate 4g	

Exchanges: 1/2 starch

Mexican Roll-Ups

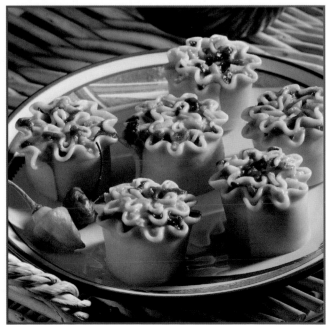

Thai-Style Pork Kabobs

(Pictured at right)

1/3 cup reduced-sodium soy sauce

2 tablespoons fresh lime juice

2 tablespoons water

2 teaspoons hot chili oil *or* 2 teaspoons canola oil plus 1/2 teaspoon crushed red pepper flakes

2 cloves garlic, minced

1 teaspoon minced fresh ginger

12 ounces well-trimmed pork tenderloin

1 medium red or yellow bell pepper, cut into 1/2-inch pieces

1 medium red or sweet onion, cut into 1/2-inch chunks

2 cups hot cooked rice

1. Combine soy sauce, lime juice, water, chili oil, garlic and ginger in medium bowl. Reserve 1/3 cup mixture for dipping sauce; set aside.

2. Cut pork tenderloin lengthwise in half; cut crosswise into 4-inch-thick slices. Cut slices into 1/2-inch strips. Add to bowl with soy sauce mixture; toss to coat. Cover; refrigerate at least 30 minutes or up to 2 hours, turning once.

3. To prevent sticking, spray grid with nonstick cooking spray. Prepare coals for grilling.

4. Remove pork from marinade; discard marinade. Alternately weave pork strips and thread bell pepper and onion chunks onto 8 (8- to 10-inch) metal skewers.

5. Grill, covered, over medium-hot coals 6 to 8 minutes or until pork is no longer pink in center, turning halfway through grilling time. Serve with rice and reserved dipping sauce.

Makes 4 servings

Nutrients per Serving: 2 Kabobs with 1/2 cup rice and about 1 tablespoon plus 1 teaspoon dipping sauce

Calories 248	**Fiber** 2g
Fat 4g (sat 1g)	**Cholesterol** 49mg
Protein 22g	**Sodium** 271mg
Carbohydrate 30g	

Exchanges: 1-1/2 starch, 1 vegetable, 2 lean meat

Spinach-Cheddar Squares

low fat low sodium

1-1/2 cups EGG BEATERS® Healthy Real Egg Product

3/4 cup fat-free (skim) milk

1 tablespoon dried onion flakes

1 tablespoon grated Parmesan cheese

1/4 teaspoon garlic powder

1/8 teaspoon ground black pepper

1/4 cup plain dry bread crumbs

3/4 cup shredded fat-free Cheddar cheese, divided

1 (10-ounce) package frozen chopped spinach, thawed and well drained

1/4 cup diced pimentos

In medium bowl, combine Egg Beaters®, milk, onion flakes, Parmesan cheese, garlic powder and pepper; set aside.

Sprinkle bread crumbs evenly onto bottom of lightly greased 8×8×2-inch baking dish. Top with 1/2 cup Cheddar cheese and spinach. Pour egg mixture evenly over spinach; top with remaining Cheddar cheese and pimentos.

Bake at 350°F for 35 to 40 minutes or until knife inserted into center comes out clean. Let stand 10 minutes before serving.

Makes 16 appetizer servings

Nutrients per Serving: 1 Square (1/16 of total recipe)

Calories 37	**Fiber** 1g
Fat <1g (sat <1g)	**Cholesterol** <1mg
Protein 5g	**Sodium** 116mg
Carbohydrate 4g	

Exchanges: 1 lean meat

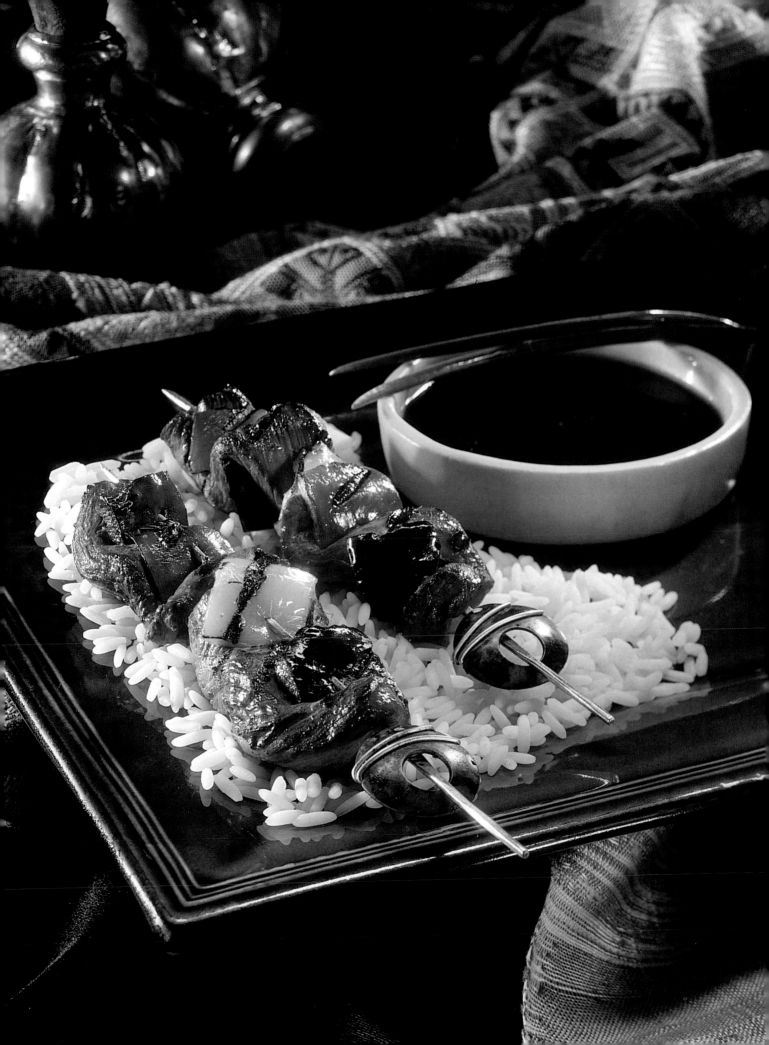

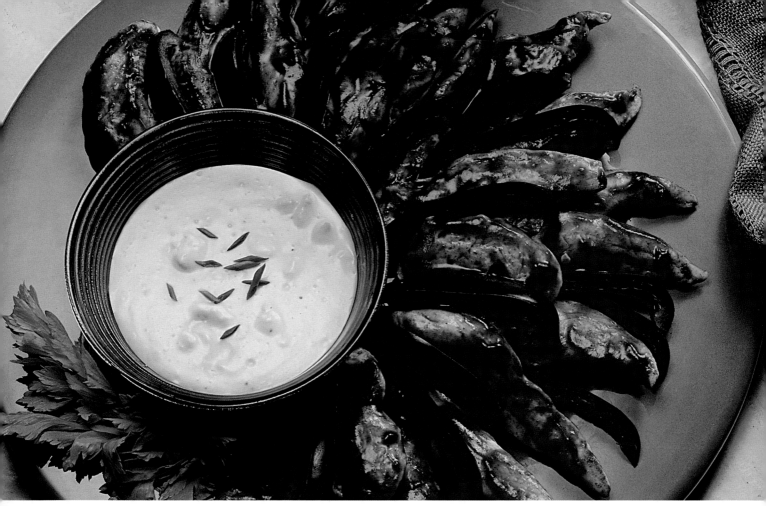

Buffalo Chicken Tenders

Buffalo Chicken Tenders

 low fat | low carb

(Pictured above)

3 tablespoons Louisiana-style hot sauce
1/2 teaspoon paprika
1/4 teaspoon ground red pepper
1 pound chicken tenders
1/2 cup fat-free blue cheese dressing
1/4 cup reduced-fat sour cream
2 tablespoons crumbled blue cheese
1 medium red bell pepper, cut into
1/2-inch slices

1. Preheat oven to 375°F. Combine hot sauce, paprika and ground red pepper in small bowl; brush on all surfaces of chicken. Place chicken in greased 11×7-inch baking dish. Cover; marinate in refrigerator 30 minutes.

2. Bake, uncovered, about 15 minutes or until chicken is no longer pink in center.

3. Combine blue cheese dressing, sour cream and blue cheese in small serving bowl. Garnish as desired. Serve with chicken and bell pepper for dipping.   *Makes 10 servings*

Nutrients per Serving: about 2 Chicken Tenders plus 1-1/2 tablespoons dipping sauce

Calories 83	**Fiber** 0g
Fat 2g (sat 1g)	**Cholesterol** 27mg
Protein 9g	**Sodium** 180mg
Carbohydrate 5g	

Exchanges: 1/2 starch, 1 lean meat

Tip

"Tenders" or "supremes" are the lean, tender strips found on the underside of the chicken breast. Skinless and boneless, these pieces are very low in fat and have virtually no waste.

Sesame Chicken Salad Wonton Cups

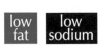

(Pictured on page 10)

Nonstick cooking spray
20 wonton wrappers (3 inches)
1 tablespoon sesame seeds
2 small boneless skinless chicken breasts
  (about 8 ounces)
1 cup fresh green beans, cut diagonally
  into 1/2-inch pieces
1/4 cup reduced-fat mayonnaise
1 tablespoon chopped fresh cilantro
  (optional)
2 teaspoons honey
1 teaspoon reduced-sodium soy sauce
1/8 teaspoon ground red pepper

1. Preheat oven to 350°F.

2. Spray miniature muffin pan with cooking spray. Press 1 wonton wrapper into each muffin cup; spray with cooking spray. Bake 8 to 10 minutes or until golden brown. Cool in pan on wire rack before filling.

3. Place sesame seeds in shallow baking pan. Bake 5 minutes or until lightly toasted, stirring occasionally. Set aside to cool.

4. Meanwhile, bring 2 cups water to a boil in medium saucepan. Add chicken. Reduce heat to low; cover. Simmer 10 minutes or until chicken is no longer pink in center; drain. In another saucepan, bring 2 cups water to a boil. Add green beans. Reduce heat to low; cover and simmer 7 minutes. Drain.

5. Finely chop chicken. Place in medium bowl. Add green beans and remaining ingredients; mix lightly. Spoon lightly rounded tablespoonful chicken mixture into each wonton cup. Garnish, if desired.   *Makes 10 servings*

Nutrients per Serving: 2 filled Wonton Cups

Calories 103	**Fiber** <1g
Fat 3g (sat 1g)	**Cholesterol** 18mg
Protein 7g	**Sodium** 128mg
Carbohydrate 12g	

Exchanges: 1 starch, 1/2 lean meat

Nutty Carrot Spread

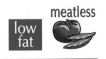

Quick Recipe   *(Pictured below)*

1/4 cup finely chopped pecans, toasted
6 ounces fat-free cream cheese, softened
2 tablespoons frozen orange juice
  concentrate, thawed
1/4 teaspoon ground cinnamon
1 cup shredded carrot
1/4 cup raisins
36 party pumpernickel bread slices,
  toasted, or melba toast rounds

1. To toast pecans, place in shallow baking pan. Bake at 350°F 10 minutes or until lightly toasted, stirring occasionally.

2. Meanwhile, combine cream cheese, orange juice concentrate and cinnamon in small bowl; stir until well blended. Stir in carrot, pecans and raisins.

3. Spread 1 tablespoon cream cheese mixture onto each bread slice. Garnish, if desired.
          Makes 18 servings

Nutrients per Serving: 2 bread slices with 2 tablespoons cream cheese mixture (1 tablespoon per bread slice)

Calories 68	**Fiber** <1g
Fat 1g (sat <1g)	**Cholesterol** 2mg
Protein 3g	**Sodium** 149mg
Carbohydrate 11g	

Exchanges: 1 starch

Nutty Carrot Spread

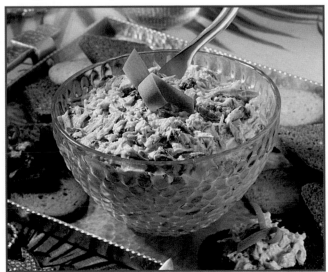

Taco Chicken Nachos

(Pictured at right)

2 boneless skinless chicken breasts (about 8 ounces)

1 tablespoon plus 1-1/2 teaspoons taco seasoning mix

1 teaspoon olive oil

3/4 cup fat-free sour cream

1 can (4 ounces) chopped mild green chilies, drained

1/4 cup minced red onion

1 bag (8 ounces) baked fat-free tortilla chips

1 cup (4 ounces) shredded reduced-fat Cheddar or Monterey Jack cheese

1/2 cup chopped fresh tomato

1/4 cup pitted ripe olive slices (optional)

2 tablespoons chopped fresh cilantro (optional)

1. Bring 2 cups water to a boil in small saucepan. Add chicken. Reduce heat to low; cover. Simmer 10 minutes or until chicken is no longer pink in center. Remove from saucepan; cool. Chop chicken.

2. Combine seasoning mix and oil in small bowl; mix until smooth paste forms. Stir in sour cream. Add chicken, green chilies and onion; mix lightly.

3. Preheat broiler. Arrange tortilla chips evenly on small ovenproof plates or large platter. Evenly cover chips with chicken mixture and cheese. Broil 4 inches from heat 2 to 3 minutes or until chicken mixture is hot and cheese is melted. Sprinkle evenly with tomato, olives and cilantro, if desired. Serve hot.

Makes 12 servings

Nutrients per Serving: about 5 tortilla chips with 3 tablespoons topping

Calories 148	**Fiber** 1g
Fat 3g (sat 1g)	**Cholesterol** 20mg
Protein 12g	**Sodium** 431mg
Carbohydrate 18g	

Exchanges: 1 starch, 1-1/2 lean meat

Angelic Deviled Eggs

6 large eggs

1/4 cup low-fat (1%) cottage cheese

3 tablespoons prepared fat-free ranch dressing

2 teaspoons Dijon mustard

2 tablespoons minced fresh chives or dill

1 tablespoon diced well-drained pimiento or roasted red pepper

1. Place eggs in medium saucepan; add enough water to cover. Bring to a boil over medium heat. Remove from heat; cover. Let stand 15 minutes. Drain. Add cold water to eggs in saucepan; let stand until eggs are cool. Drain. Remove shells from eggs; discard shells.

2. Cut eggs lengthwise in half. Remove yolks, reserving 3 yolk halves. Discard remaining yolks or reserve for another use. Place egg whites, cut sides up, on serving plate; cover with plastic wrap. Refrigerate while preparing filling.

3. Combine cottage cheese, dressing, mustard and reserved yolk halves in mini food processor; process until smooth. (Or, place in small bowl and mash with fork until well blended.) Transfer cheese mixture to small bowl; stir in chives and pimiento. Evenly spoon into egg whites. Cover and chill at least 1 hour. Garnish, if desired.

Makes 12 servings

Nutrients per Serving: 1 filled Egg half

Calories 24	**Fiber** 1g
Fat 1g (sat <1g)	**Cholesterol** 27mg
Protein 3g	**Sodium** 96mg
Carbohydrate 1g	

Exchanges: 1/2 lean meat

Taco Chicken Nachos

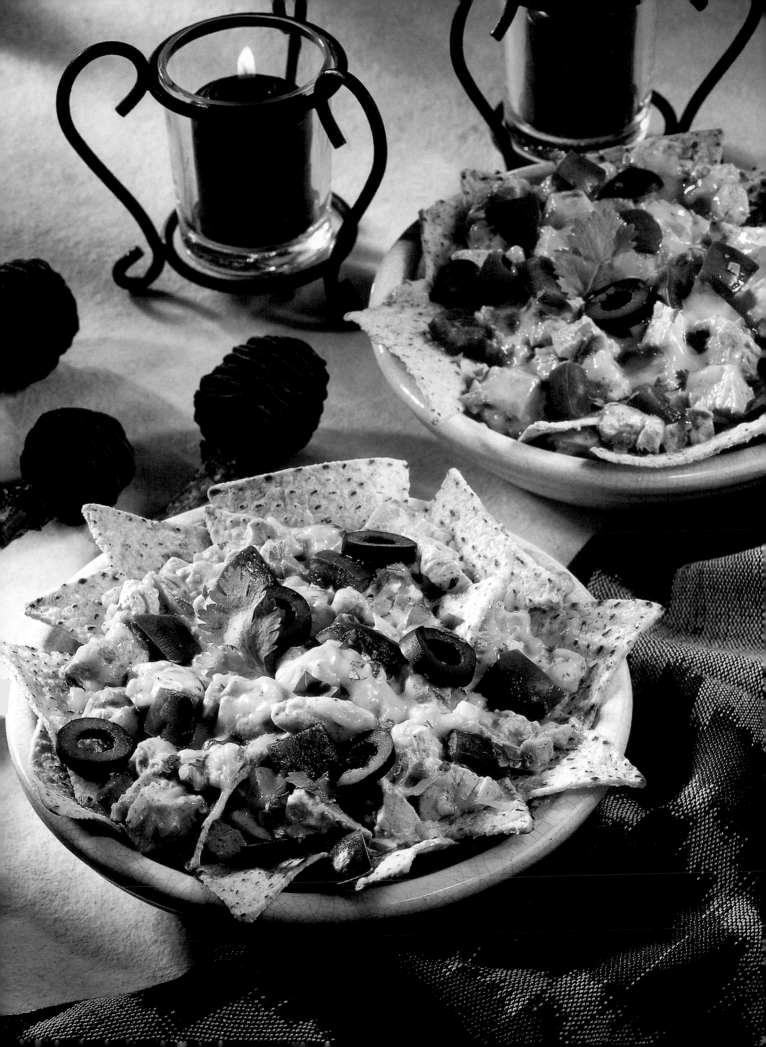

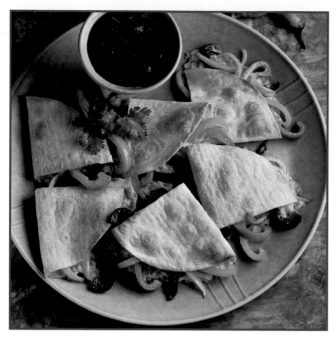

Cheesy Pepper & Onion Quesadillas

Cheesy Pepper & Onion Quesadillas

 meatless

Quick Recipe   (Pictured above)

1/3 cup margarine
3-3/4 cups frozen stir-fry vegetable blend (onions and red, yellow and green bell peppers)
3/4 teaspoon chili powder
1 package (8 ounces) fat-free cream cheese, softened
1 package (8 ounces) shredded fat-free Cheddar cheese
10 flour tortillas (6 inches)
Salsa (optional)

1. Preheat oven to 425°F. Heat margarine in large nonstick skillet over medium heat until melted. Add stir-fry blend and chili powder. Cook and stir until tender. Drain, reserving margarine.

2. Beat cream cheese with electric mixer on medium speed until smooth. Add Cheddar cheese, mixing until blended. Spread 2 tablespoons cheese mixture onto each tortilla; top with pepper mixture. Fold tortillas in half; place on baking sheet. Brush with reserved margarine.

3. Bake 10 minutes. Cut each tortilla in half. Serve warm with salsa, if desired.

Makes 20 appetizers

Nutrients per Serving: 1 Quesadilla half (1/2 of filled tortilla)

Calories 118	**Fiber** 1g
Fat 4g (sat 1g)	**Cholesterol** 1mg
Protein 7g	**Sodium** 266mg
Carbohydrate 12g	

Exchanges: 1/2 starch, 1 vegetable, 1 fat

❧ ❧ ❧

Pinwheel Appetizers

 low fat | low sodium | low carb

3 cups cooked wild rice
1 package (8 ounces) fat-free pasteurized process cream cheese product
1/3 cup grated Parmesan cheese
1 teaspoon dried parsley flakes
1/2 teaspoon garlic powder
1/2 teaspoon Dijon-style mustard
2 to 3 drops hot pepper sauce (optional)
3 soft flour tortillas (10 inches)
2-1/2 ounces thinly sliced corned beef
9 fresh spinach leaves

Combine wild rice, cream cheese, Parmesan cheese, parsley, garlic powder, mustard and pepper sauce. Spread evenly over tortillas, leaving 1/2-inch border on one side of each tortilla. Place single layer corned beef over rice and cheese mixture. Top with layer of spinach. Roll each tortilla tightly toward 1/2-inch border. Moisten border of tortilla with water; press to seal roll. Wrap tightly in plastic wrap. Refrigerate several hours or overnight. Cut into 1-inch slices. *Makes 36 appetizers*

Favorite recipe from **Minnesota Cultivated Wild Rice Council**

Nutrients per Serving: 1 Pinwheel Appetizer

Calories 37	**Fiber** <1g
Fat 1g (sat <1g)	**Cholesterol** 4mg
Protein 2g	**Sodium** 91mg
Carbohydrate 5g	

Exchanges: 1/2 starch

Festive Crab Toasts

Quick Recipe

- **12 ounces crabmeat, flaked**
- **1 can (10-3/4 ounces) reduced-fat condensed cream of celery soup, undiluted**
- **1/4 cup chopped celery**
- **1/4 cup sliced green onions**
- **1 tablespoon fresh lemon juice**
- **1/8 teaspoon grated lemon peel**
- **1 French bread baguette (8 ounces)**
- **1/3 cup grated Parmesan cheese**
  Paprika

1. Combine crabmeat, soup, celery, onions, lemon juice and lemon peel in medium bowl; mix well. Cut baguette diagonally into 1/2-inch-thick slices; arrange slices on 2 ungreased baking sheets. Broil 5 inches from heat 2 minutes or until toasted, turning once.

2. Spread 1 tablespoon crab mixture onto each baguette slice. Top with Parmesan cheese; sprinkle with paprika. Broil 5 inches from heat 2 minutes or until lightly browned.

Makes about 30 appetizers

Nutrients per Serving: 1 Crab Toast

Calories 44	**Fiber** <1g
Fat 1g (sat <1g)	**Cholesterol** 11mg
Protein 4g	**Sodium** 182mg
Carbohydrate 5g	

Exchanges: 1/2 starch

Mini Marinated Beef Skewers

(Pictured at right)

- **1 pound lean beef round tip, cut 1 inch thick**
- **2 tablespoons reduced-sodium soy sauce**
- **1 tablespoon dry sherry or apple juice**
- **1 teaspoon dark sesame oil**
- **2 cloves garlic, minced**
- **18 cherry tomatoes (optional)**

1. Cut beef across the grain into 1/8-inch slices. Place in large resealable plastic food storage bag. Combine soy sauce, sherry or juice, oil and garlic in cup; pour over steak. Seal bag; turn to coat. Marinate in refrigerator at least 30 minutes or up to 2 hours.

2. Soak 18 (6-inch) wooden skewers in water 20 minutes.

3. Drain steak; discard marinade. Weave beef accordion-fashion onto skewers. Place on rack of broiler pan. Broil 4 to 5 inches from heat 2 minutes. Turn skewers over; broil 2 minutes or until beef is barely pink.

4. Garnish each skewer with 1 cherry tomato, if desired. Place skewers on lettuce-lined platter. Serve warm.

Makes 6 servings (3 skewers each)

Nutrients per Serving: 3 Skewers (without lettuce)

Calories 120	**Fiber** <1g
Fat 4g (sat 1g)	**Cholesterol** 60mg
Protein 20g	**Sodium** 99mg
Carbohydrate 2g	

Exchanges: 2 lean meat

Mini Marinated Beef Skewers

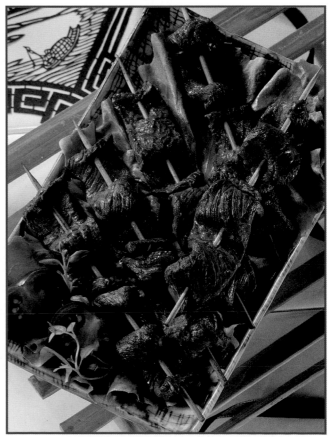

Grilled Red Bell Pepper Dip

(Pictured at right)

1 medium red bell pepper, halved and seeded
1 cup fat-free or reduced-fat ricotta cheese
4 ounces fat-free cream cheese
1/4 cup (1 ounce) grated Parmesan cheese
1 clove Grilled Garlic (recipe follows) *or* 1 clove garlic, minced
1/2 teaspoon Dijon mustard
1/4 teaspoon salt
1/4 teaspoon herbes de Provence*
Mini pita pockets, Melba toast, pretzels or fresh vegetables (optional)

Substitute dash each rubbed sage, crushed dried rosemary, thyme, oregano, marjoram and basil leaves for herbes de Provence.

1. Grill bell pepper halves skin-side down on covered grill over medium coals 15 to 25 minutes or until skin is charred, without turning. Remove from grill and immediately place in bowl; cover and let stand 15 to 20 minutes. Remove skin with paring knife; discard.

2. Place bell pepper in food processor. Add cheeses, garlic, mustard, salt and herbes de Provence; process until smooth. Serve with mini pita pockets or vegetables for dipping, if desired.   *Makes about 2 cups dip*

Grilled Garlic

2 cloves garlic
Nonstick cooking spray

Thread garlic cloves onto water-soaked wooden or bamboo skewer. Spray with cooking spray. Grill on covered or uncovered grill over medium coals about 8 minutes or until browned and tender. Or, place 2 garlic cloves on sheet of foil; lightly spray with cooking spray and carefully seal foil packet. Finish grilling as directed.

Nutrients per Serving: 2 tablespoons Dip

Calories 26	**Fiber** <1g
Fat 1g (sat <1g)	**Cholesterol** 3mg
Protein 4g	**Sodium** 130mg
Carbohydrate 1g	

Exchanges: 1/2 lean meat

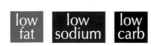

Savory Zucchini Stix

Olive oil-flavored nonstick cooking spray
3 tablespoons seasoned dry bread crumbs
2 tablespoons grated Parmesan cheese
1 egg white
1 teaspoon 2% milk
2 small zucchini (about 4 ounces each), cut lengthwise into quarters
1/3 cup spaghetti sauce, warmed

1. Preheat oven to 400°F. Spray baking sheet with cooking spray; set aside.

2. Combine bread crumbs and Parmesan cheese in shallow dish. Combine egg white and milk in another shallow dish; beat with fork until well blended.

3. Dip each zucchini wedge first into crumb mixture, then into egg white mixture, letting excess drip back into dish. Roll again in crumb mixture to coat.

4. Place zucchini sticks on prepared baking sheet; coat well with cooking spray. Bake 15 to 18 minutes or until golden brown. Serve with spaghetti sauce.   *Makes 4 servings*

Nutrients per Serving: 2 Stix with 1 tablespoon plus 1 teaspoon spaghetti sauce

Calories 69	**Fiber** 1g
Fat 2g (sat 1g)	**Cholesterol** 6mg
Protein 4g	**Sodium** 329mg
Carbohydrate 9g	

Exchanges: 2 vegetable, 1/2 fat

Grilled Red Bell Pepper Dip

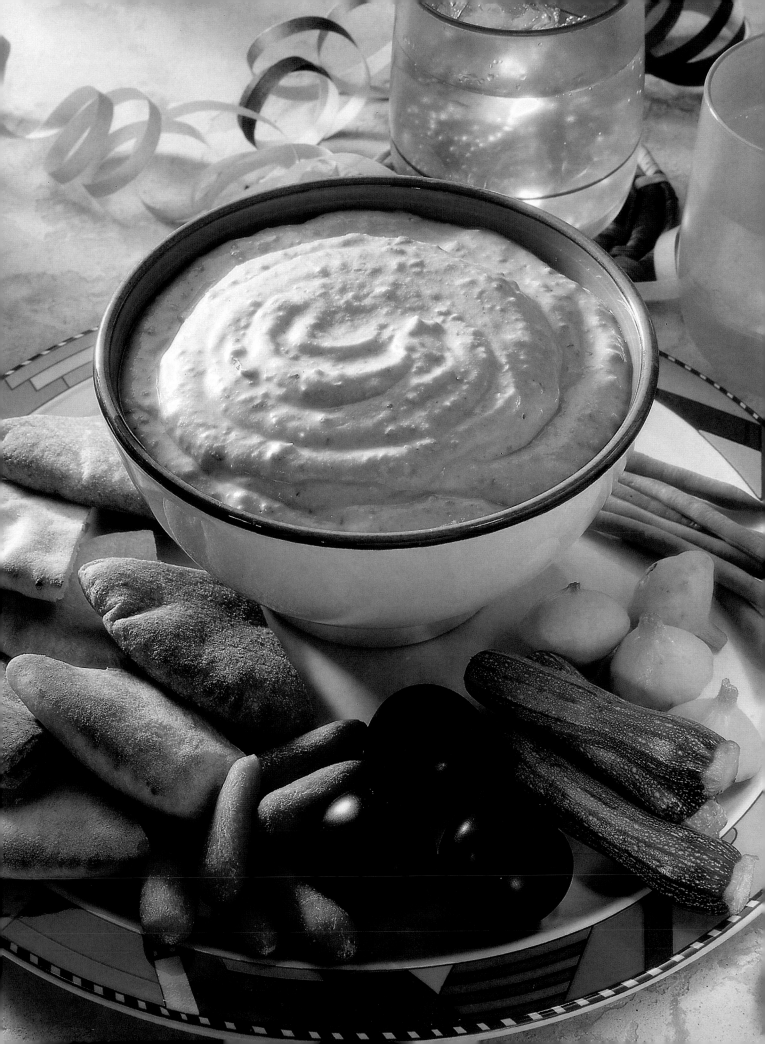

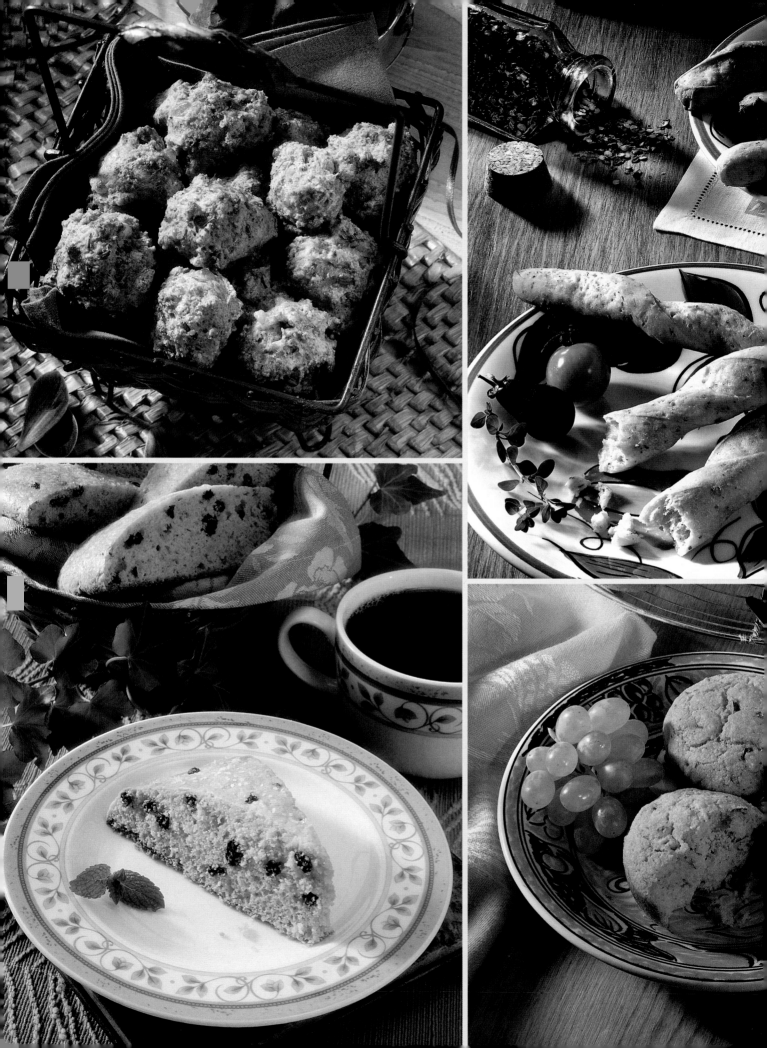

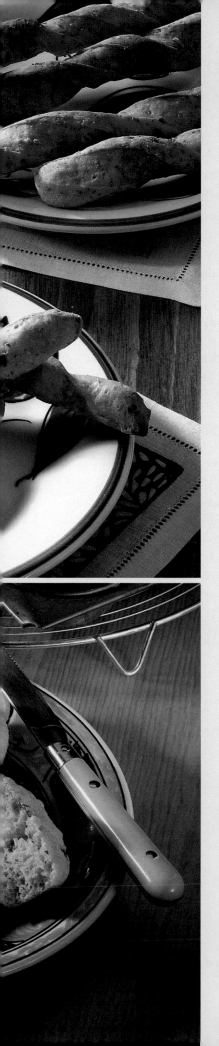

Breads

❧ ❧ ❧

Spicy Corn Muffins

Quick Recipe   *(Pictured at left)*

> 1 cup low-fat buttermilk
> 1 tablespoon vegetable oil
> 1 egg white
> 1 serrano or other hot pepper,* minced
> 1 cup cornmeal
> 1/3 cup all-purpose flour
> 1 tablespoon finely chopped fresh cilantro or parsley
> 1 teaspoon baking powder
> 1/2 teaspoon baking soda
> 1/4 teaspoon salt
> 1/4 teaspoon ground cumin
> 1/4 teaspoon ground paprika

*Serrano peppers can sting and irritate the skin; wear rubber gloves when handling peppers and do not touch eyes. Wash hands after handling peppers.

1. Preheat oven to 400°F. Spray 6-cup muffin pan with nonstick cooking spray; set aside.

2. Combine buttermilk, oil, egg white and serrano pepper in small bowl until smooth. Combine cornmeal, flour, cilantro, baking powder, baking soda, salt, cumin and paprika in medium bowl; mix well. Make well in dry ingredients; pour in buttermilk mixture. Stir with fork just until dry ingredients are moistened.

3. Spoon batter evenly into prepared muffin cups. Bake 15 to 20 minutes or until toothpick inserted into centers comes out clean.   *Makes 6 muffins*

Nutrients per Serving: 1 Muffin

Calories 140	**Fiber** 3g
Fat 3g (sat 1g)	**Cholesterol** 2mg
Protein 4g	**Sodium** 308mg
Carbohydrate 23g	

Exchanges: 1-1/2 starch, 1/2 fat

Clockwise from top left: Chive Whole Wheat Drop Biscuits (page 39), Pizza Breadsticks (page 39), Spicy Corn Muffins, and Cornmeal Scones (page 51)

Apple Streusel Mini Muffins

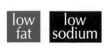

Quick Recipe   *(Pictured at right)*

1/4 cup chopped pecans
2 tablespoons brown sugar
1 tablespoon all-purpose flour
2 teaspoons butter, melted
1 package (7 ounces) apple-cinnamon muffin mix
1/2 cup shredded peeled apple

1. Preheat oven to 425°F. Coat 18 mini-muffin cups with nonstick cooking spray; set aside.

2. Combine pecans, brown sugar, flour and butter in small bowl.

3. Prepare muffin mix according to package directions. Stir in apple. Fill each muffin cup 2/3 full. Sprinkle approximately 1 teaspoon pecan mixture on top of each muffin.

4. Bake 12 to 15 minutes or until golden brown. Cool slightly. Serve warm.

Makes 18 mini muffins

Nutrients per Serving: 1 Mini Muffin

Calories 77	**Fiber** 1g
Fat 3g (sat 1g)	**Cholesterol** 1mg
Protein 1g	**Sodium** 90mg
Carbohydrate 10g	

Exchanges: 1 starch

Tip

Toast the pecans for extra flavor. Spread them evenly in a small baking pan, and bake them in a 400°F oven 5 to 7 minutes or until light golden brown. Or, spread the nuts on a plate and microwave them on HIGH 1 minute. Stir them, then continue microwaving, checking every 30 seconds, until the pecans are crunchy.

Irish Potato Soda Bread

1 medium COLORADO potato, peeled and coarsely chopped
1/2 cup water
1/4 cup buttermilk
2 cups all-purpose flour
1 teaspoon baking powder
1/2 teaspoon baking soda
1/4 teaspoon salt
1/4 cup cold butter
2 eggs, beaten, divided
1/3 cup dried currants or raisins

In small saucepan cook potato and water, covered, over medium heat about 10 minutes or until tender. *Do not drain.* Mash until smooth or place mixture in blender; blend until smooth. Add buttermilk to measure 1 cup. In mixing bowl combine flour, baking powder, baking soda and salt. Cut in butter until mixture resembles coarse crumbs. Combine potato mixture, 1 beaten egg and currants; add to flour mixture. Stir until dough clings together. Stir mixture vigorously in bowl 12 to 15 strokes; form into ball. Turn ball of dough out onto lightly greased baking sheet. With sharp knife make a 4-inch cross, 1/4 inch deep, on top of loaf. Brush with remaining beaten egg. Bake in 375°F oven about 35 minutes or until golden. Cool on wire rack.   *Makes 16 servings*

Favorite recipe from **Colorado Potato Administrative Committee**

Nutrients per Serving: 1 slice (1/16 of loaf)

Calories 111	**Fiber** 1g
Fat 4g (sat 2g)	**Cholesterol** 35mg
Protein 3g	**Sodium** 150mg
Carbohydrate 16g	

Exchanges: 1 starch, 1 fat

Apple Streusel Mini Muffins

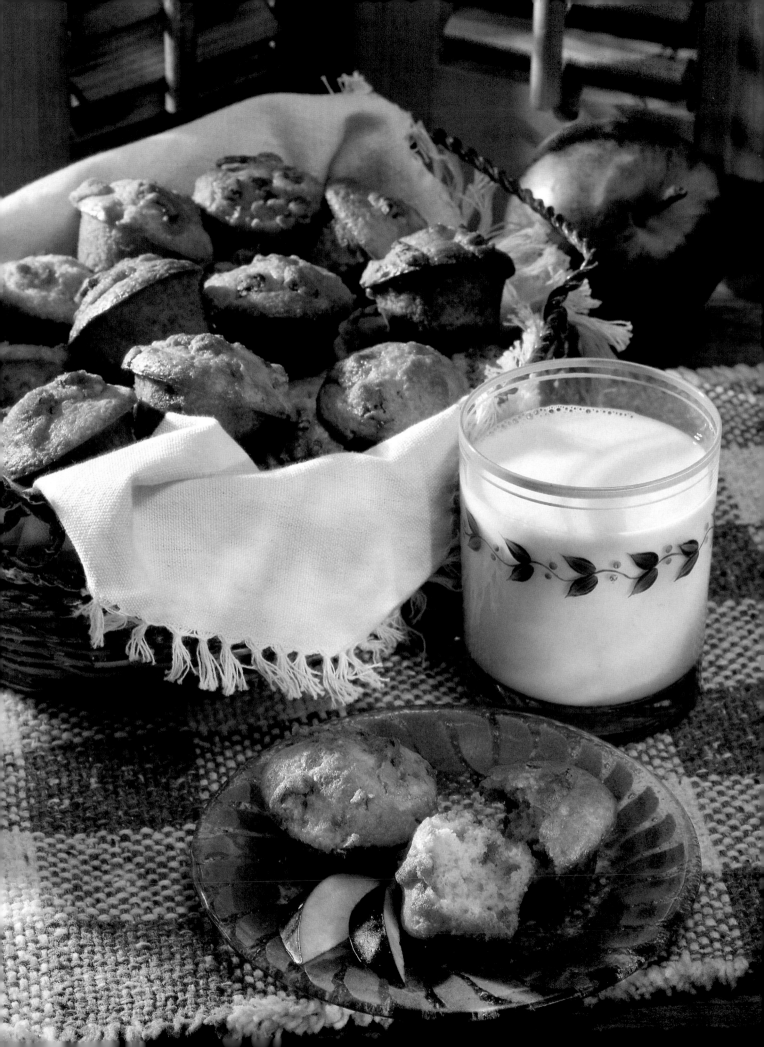

Whole Wheat Herb Bread

(Pictured at right)

2/3 cup water

2/3 cup fat-free milk

2 teaspoons sugar

2 packages (1/4 ounce each) active dry yeast

3 egg whites, lightly beaten

3 tablespoons olive oil

1 teaspoon salt

1/2 teaspoon dried basil leaves

1/2 teaspoon dried oregano leaves

4 to 4-1/2 cups whole wheat flour, divided

1. Bring water to a boil in small saucepan. Remove from heat; stir in milk and sugar. When mixture is warm (110° to 115°F), add yeast. Mix well; let stand 10 minutes or until bubbly.

2. Combine egg whites, oil, salt, basil and oregano in large bowl until well blended. Add yeast mixture; mix well. Add 4 cups flour, 1/2 cup at a time, mixing well after each addition, until dough is no longer sticky. Knead about 5 minutes or until smooth and elastic, adding enough of remaining flour to make a smooth and elastic dough. Form into a ball. Cover and let rise in warm place about 1 hour or until doubled in bulk.

3. Preheat oven to 350°F. Punch dough down and place on lightly floured surface. Divide evenly into 4 pieces and roll each piece into a ball. Lightly spray baking sheet with nonstick cooking spray. Place dough balls on prepared baking sheet. Bake 30 to 35 minutes or until golden brown and loaves sound hollow when tapped with finger. *Makes 24 servings (4 round loaves, 6 slices per loaf)*

Nutrients per Serving: 1 slice (1/6 of 1 round loaf)

Calories 90	**Fiber** 3g
Fat 2g (sat <1g)	**Cholesterol** <1mg
Protein 4g	**Sodium** 109mg
Carbohydrate 17g	

Exchanges: 1 starch

Focaccia

3/4 cup warm water (110° to 115°F)

1-1/2 teaspoons sugar

1 teaspoon active dry yeast

1 tablespoon extra-virgin olive oil

1 teaspoon salt

1 teaspoon dried rosemary leaves, crushed

1 cup all-purpose flour

1 cup whole wheat flour

Nonstick cooking spray

1. Pour water into large bowl. Dissolve sugar and yeast in water; let stand 10 minutes or until bubbly. Stir in oil, salt and rosemary. Add flours, 1/2 cup at a time, stirring until dough begins to pull away from side of bowl and form a ball.

2. Turn dough out onto lightly floured surface and knead 5 minutes or until dough is smooth and elastic, adding more flour if necessary. Place dough in bowl lightly sprayed with cooking spray and turn dough so all sides are coated. Cover with towel or plastic wrap and let rise in warm, draft-free place about 1 hour or until doubled in bulk.

3. Turn dough out onto lightly floured surface and knead 1 minute. Divide evenly into 3 balls; roll each into 6-inch circle. Using fingertips, dimple surfaces of dough. Place on baking sheet sprayed with cooking spray; cover and let rise 30 minutes more.

4. Preheat oven to 400°F. Spray tops of dough circles with cooking spray; bake about 13 minutes or until golden brown. Remove from oven and cut each loaf into 10 wedges.

Makes 10 servings (30 wedges)

Nutrients per Serving: 3 wedges (1/10 of total recipe)

Calories 102	**Fiber** 2g
Fat 2g (sat <1g)	**Cholesterol** 0mg
Protein 3g	**Sodium** 214mg
Carbohydrate 19g	

Exchanges: 1-1/2 starch

Whole Wheat Herb Bread

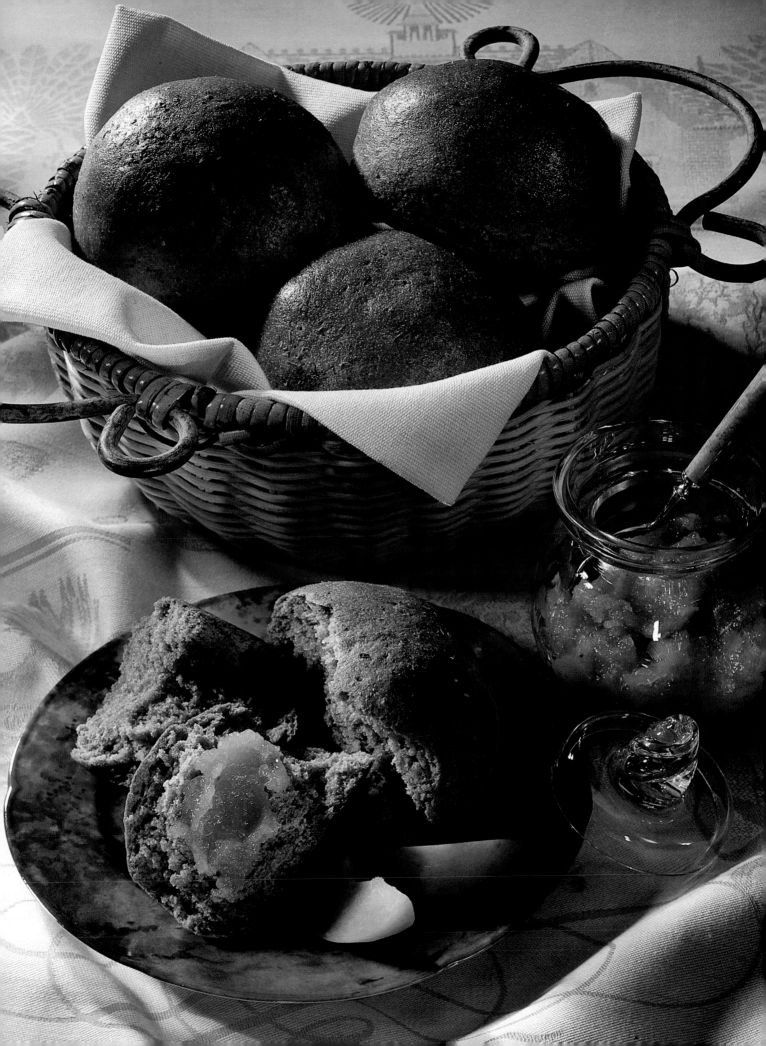

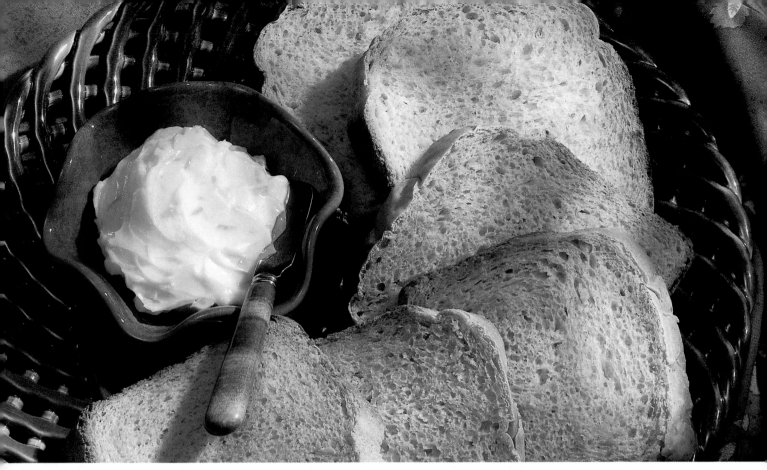

Multigrain Bread

Multigrain Bread

(Pictured above)

1-1/2-POUND LOAF
  1-1/4 cups boiling water
   1/4 cup multigrain cereal
    2 tablespoons uncooked quick oats
    2 tablespoons honey
    1 tablespoon margarine or butter
    1 teaspoon salt
  2-1/2 cups bread flour
  1-1/2 teaspoons rapid-rise yeast

2-POUND LOAF
  1-1/2 cups boiling water
   1/3 cup multigrain cereal
   1/4 cup uncooked quick oats
    3 tablespoons honey
  1-1/2 tablespoons margarine or butter
  1-1/2 teaspoons salt
  3-1/4 cups bread flour
    2 teaspoons rapid-rise yeast

1. Measuring carefully, place water in bread machine pan. Add cereal and oats. Let stand 30 minutes or until cool. Add remaining ingredients in order specified by owner's manual.

2. Program basic cycle and desired crust setting; press start.

3. Remove baked bread from pan; cool on wire rack.   *Makes 12 or 16 servings*

Nutrients per Serving: 1 slice (1/12 of 1-1/2-pound loaf)

Calories 132	**Fiber** 1g
Fat 2g (sat <1g)	**Cholesterol** 0mg
Protein 4g	**Sodium** 206mg
Carbohydrate 26g	

Exchanges: 1-1/2 starch

Chive Whole Wheat Drop Biscuits

Quick Recipe   *(Pictured on page 32)*

 1-1/4 cups whole wheat flour
   3/4 cup all-purpose flour
      3 tablespoons toasted wheat germ, divided
      1 tablespoon baking powder
      1 tablespoon chopped fresh chives *or* 1 teaspoon dried chives
      2 teaspoons sugar
      3 tablespoons cold margarine
      1 cup fat-free milk
   1/2 cup (2 ounces) shredded low-fat process American cheese

1. Preheat oven to 450°F. Spray baking sheet with nonstick cooking spray; set aside.

2. Combine whole wheat flour, all-purpose flour, 2 tablespoons wheat germ, baking powder, chives and sugar in medium bowl. Cut in margarine with pastry blender or two knives until mixture resembles coarse meal. Add milk and American cheese; stir until just combined.

3. Drop dough by rounded teaspoonfuls onto prepared baking sheet about 1 inch apart. Sprinkle with remaining 1 tablespoon wheat germ.

4. Bake 10 to 12 minutes or until golden brown. Remove immediately from baking sheet. Serve warm.   *Makes 12 servings*

Nutrients per Serving: 1 Biscuit

Calories 125	**Fiber** 2g
Fat 4g (sat 2g)	**Cholesterol** 3mg
Protein 5g	**Sodium** 237mg
Carbohydrate 18g	

Exchanges: 1 starch, 1 fat

Pizza Breadsticks

low fat   low sodium

(Pictured on page 32)

      1 package (1/4 ounce) active dry yeast
   3/4 cup warm water (105° to 115°F)
 2-1/2 cups all-purpose flour
   1/2 cup (2 ounces) shredded part-skim mozzarella cheese
   1/4 cup (1 ounce) shredded Parmesan cheese
   1/4 cup chopped red bell pepper
      1 green onion with top, sliced
      1 medium clove garlic, minced
   1/2 teaspoon dried basil leaves, crushed
   1/2 teaspoon dried oregano leaves, crushed
   1/4 teaspoon salt
   1/4 teaspoon red pepper flakes (optional)
      1 tablespoon olive oil

1. Preheat oven to 400°F. Spray 2 large nonstick baking sheets with nonstick cooking spray; set aside. Sprinkle yeast over warm water in small bowl; stir until yeast dissolves. Let stand 5 minutes or until bubbly.

2. Meanwhile, place all remaining ingredients except olive oil in food processor; process a few seconds to combine. With food processor running, gradually add yeast mixture and olive oil. Process just until mixture forms a ball. (Add an additional 2 tablespoons flour if dough is too sticky.)

3. Transfer dough to lightly floured surface; knead 1 minute. Let dough rest 5 minutes. Roll out dough with lightly floured rolling pin to form 14×8-inch rectangle; cut dough crosswise into 1/2-inch-wide strips. Twist dough strips; place on prepared baking sheets. Bake 14 to 16 minutes or until lightly browned.
                        Makes 14 servings

Nutrients per Serving: 2 Breadsticks

Calories 112	**Fiber** 1g
Fat 2g (sat 1g)	**Cholesterol** 4mg
Protein 4g	**Sodium** 91mg
Carbohydrate 18g	

Exchanges: 1 starch, 1/2 fat

Swedish Limpa Bread

low fat

(Pictured at right)

1-3/4 to 2 cups all-purpose flour, divided
1/2 cup rye flour
1 package (1/4 ounce) active dry yeast
1 tablespoon sugar
1-1/2 teaspoons grated orange peel
1 teaspoon salt
1/2 teaspoon fennel seeds, crushed
1/2 teaspoon caraway seeds, crushed
3/4 cup plus 4 teaspoons water, divided
4 tablespoons molasses, divided
2 tablespoons margarine or butter
1 teaspoon instant coffee granules
1/4 teaspoon whole fennel seeds
1/4 teaspoon whole caraway seeds

1. Combine 1-1/2 cups all-purpose flour, rye flour, yeast, sugar, orange peel, salt and crushed fennel and caraway seeds in large bowl.

2. Heat 3/4 cup water, 3 tablespoons molasses and margarine in small saucepan over low heat until temperature reaches 120° to 130°F. Stir in coffee.

3. Stir water mixture into flour mixture with rubber spatula to form soft but sticky dough. Gradually add more all-purpose flour to form rough dough.

4. Turn out dough onto lightly floured surface. Knead 2 minutes or until soft dough forms, gradually adding remaining flour to prevent sticking, if necessary. Cover with inverted bowl; let rest 5 minutes.

5. Continue kneading 5 to 8 minutes or until smooth and elastic. Shape dough into a ball; place in large bowl sprayed with nonstick cooking spray. Turn dough over so top is coated with cooking spray. Loosely cover with lightly greased sheet of plastic wrap. Let rise in warm place 75 minutes or until almost doubled in bulk.

6. Punch down dough. Spray 8-1/2×4-1/2-inch loaf pan with nonstick cooking spray. Roll dough into 12×7-inch rectangle. Starting with one short end, roll up tightly, jelly-roll style. Pinch seams and ends to seal. Place seam-side down in prepared pan. Cover loosely with plastic wrap. Let rise in warm place 1 hour or until doubled in bulk.

7. Preheat oven to 350°F. Stir remaining 1 tablespoon molasses and 4 teaspoons water in small bowl; set aside.

8. Uncover loaf; using sharp knife, make 3 diagonal slashes on top of dough. Bake 40 to 45 minutes or until loaf sounds hollow when tapped. Brush top with molasses mixture and sprinkle with whole fennel and caraway seeds halfway through baking time. Brush again with molasses mixture about 10 minutes before removing loaf from oven.

9. Remove from oven. Cool in pan on wire rack 5 minutes. Remove from pan. Cool completely on wire rack. *Makes 12 servings*

Nutrients per Serving: 1 slice (1/12 of loaf) without butter hearts

Calories 123	**Fiber** 1g
Fat 2g (sat <1g)	**Cholesterol** 0mg
Protein 3g	**Sodium** 219mg
Carbohydrate 23g	

Exchanges: 1-1/2 starch, 1/2 fat

Tip

Knead bread dough on a lightly floured surface. Always use the heel of your hand to knead, not your fingers. Push the dough away from you with the heel of your hand, then bring the far end down to fold the dough in half. Give the dough a quarter turn and repeat the process, adding more flour as needed to prevent sticking. You should develop a rhythm to your kneading, making the motion fluid and continuous. Knead the dough eight to ten minutes or until it is smooth and satiny and springs back when pressed with your finger.

Swedish Limpa Bread

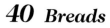

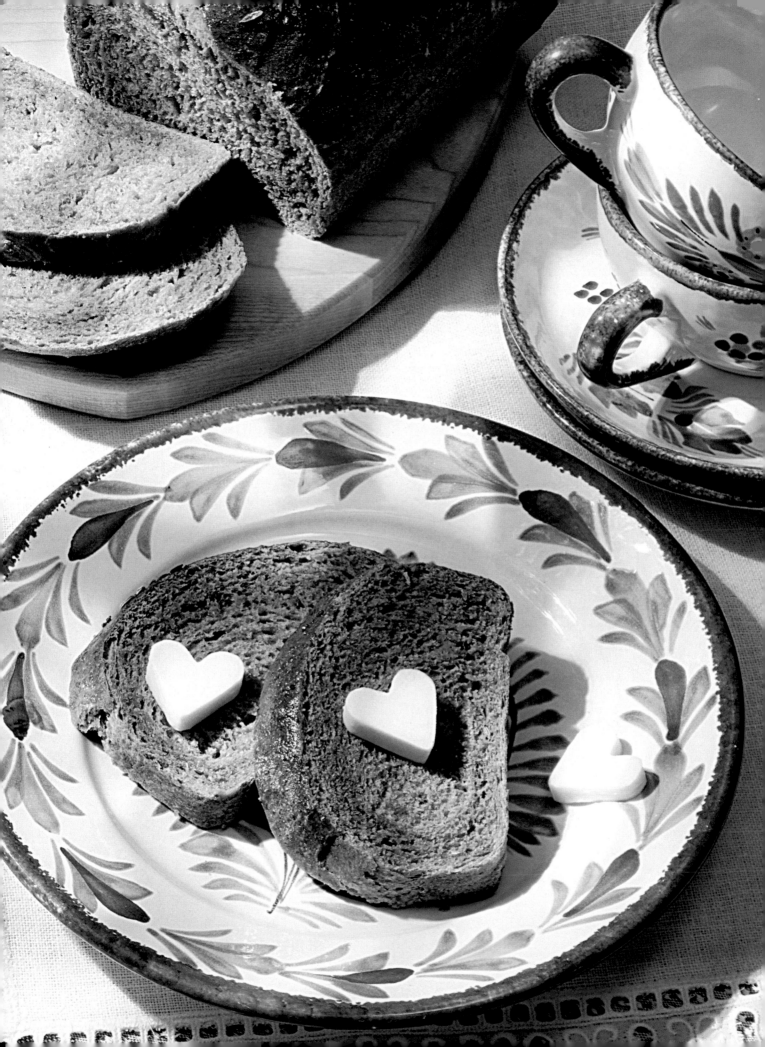

Dilled Buttermilk Bread

(Pictured at right)

1-1/2-POUND LOAF

1/2 cup water
1 egg, lightly beaten
1/2 cup buttermilk*
1 tablespoon butter
1 teaspoon salt
3 cups bread flour
1 tablespoon sugar
1-1/2 teaspoons dried dill weed
1-1/2 teaspoons rapid-rise active dry yeast

2-POUND LOAF

3/4 cup water
1 egg, lightly beaten
3/4 cup buttermilk*
1-1/2 tablespoons butter
1-1/2 teaspoons salt
4 cups bread flour
2 tablespoons sugar
2 teaspoons dried dill weed
2 teaspoons rapid-rise active dry yeast

You may substitute soured fresh milk. To sour milk, place 1 tablespoon lemon juice plus enough milk to equal 1 cup in 2-cup measure. Stir; let stand 5 minutes before using.

1. Measuring carefully, place all ingredients in bread machine pan in order specified by owner's manual.

2. Program basic cycle and desired crust setting; press start. *(Do not use delay cycles.)* Remove baked bread from pan; cool on wire rack.

Makes 12 servings

Nutrients per Serving: 1 slice (1/12 of 1-1/2-pound loaf)

Calories 149	**Fiber** 1g
Fat 2g (sat 1g)	**Cholesterol** 21mg
Protein 5g	**Sodium** 221mg
Carbohydrate 27g	

Exchanges: 2 starch

Peppered Parmesan Breadsticks

1 cup warm water (105° to 115°F)
1 package active dry yeast
1 tablespoon sugar
1 cup FIBER ONE® cereal
2-1/4 cups GOLD MEDAL® all-purpose flour
1/2 cup shredded Parmesan cheese
1-1/2 teaspoons grated lemon peel
1 teaspoon garlic salt
1 teaspoon coarsely ground black pepper
1/4 to 1/2 teaspoon ground red pepper (cayenne)
2 tablespoons olive oil
Cornmeal
1 egg white, slightly beaten

1. Stir together water, yeast and sugar. Let stand 5 minutes. Crush cereal.* Place cereal, flour, cheese, lemon peel, garlic salt and peppers in food processor. Cover and process about 10 seconds or until blended. Add oil; cover and process 10 seconds longer. Add yeast mixture; cover and process, using quick on-and-off motions, until dough forms a ball. Let rest 5 minutes. Cover and process 10 seconds. Remove dough; cover and let rise 10 minutes.

2. Heat oven to 325°F. Spray 2 cookie sheets with cooking spray. Divide dough into 16 equal parts. Roll each part into thin rope about 14 inches long on surface sprinkled with cornmeal. Place on cookie sheets. Brush with egg white; sprinkle with additional ground black and red peppers, if desired. Let stand 15 minutes.

3. Bake 25 to 35 minutes or until golden brown. Cool on wire rack. *Makes 16 breadsticks*

Place cereal in plastic bag or between sheets of waxed paper and crush with rolling pin.

Nutrients per Serving: 1 Breadstick

Calories 104	**Fiber** 3g
Fat 3g (sat <1g)	**Cholesterol** 2mg
Protein 4g	**Sodium** 195mg
Carbohydrate 18g	

Exchanges: 1 starch, 1/2 fat

Dilled Buttermilk Bread

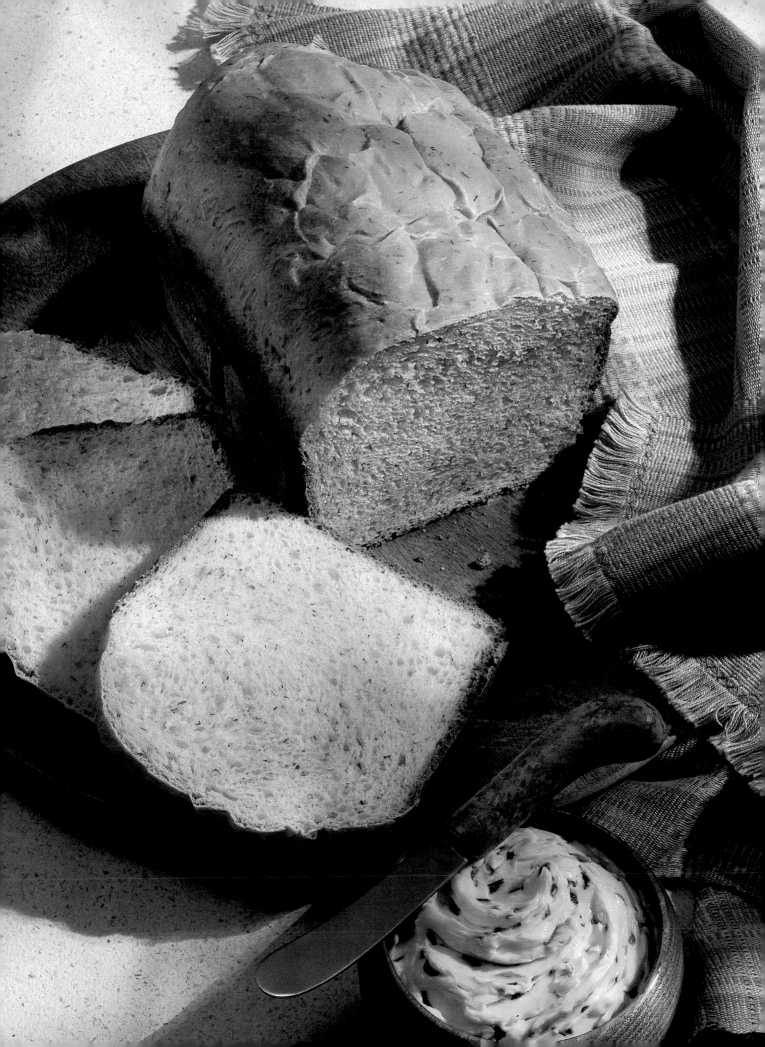

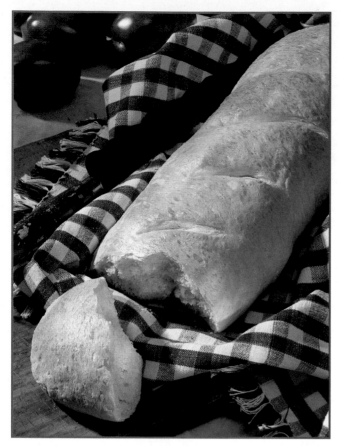

Italian Bread

Italian Bread

(Pictured above)

- **1 cup plus 2 tablespoons water, divided**
- **3 to 3-1/2 cups all-purpose flour, divided**
- **1 package (1/4 ounce) active dry yeast**
- **1 teaspoon sugar**
- **3/4 teaspoon salt**
- **1 teaspoon cornmeal**
- **1 egg**

1. Heat 1 cup water in small saucepan over low heat until temperature reaches 120° to 130°F.

2. Combine 2 cups flour, yeast, sugar and salt in large bowl. Stir heated water into flour mixture with rubber spatula to form soft dough. Gradually add about 1 cup flour, stirring 2 minutes or until dough begins to lose its stickiness.

3. Turn out dough onto lightly floured surface. Knead 5 to 8 minutes or until smooth and elastic, gradually adding remaining flour to prevent sticking, if necessary. Shape dough into a ball; place in bowl sprayed with nonstick cooking spray. Turn dough over so top is coated with cooking spray. Cover loosely with plastic wrap; let rise in warm place 1 hour or until doubled in bulk.

4. Punch down dough. Gently flatten into 10-inch circle. Starting with one side, roll up tightly, jelly-roll style. Pinch seams and ends to seal. Taper ends gently by rolling back and forth. (Finished loaf should be about 12 inches long.)

5. Spray large cookie sheet with nonstick cooking spray; sprinkle lightly with cornmeal. Place loaf on cookie sheet, seam side down. Loosely cover with lightly greased piece of plastic wrap. Let rise in warm place 30 to 40 minutes or until almost doubled in bulk.

6. Preheat oven to 350°F. Beat egg and remaining 2 tablespoons water in small bowl.

7. Uncover loaf. Using sharp knife, cut 4 or 5 diagonal slashes, each about 3 inches long, in top of loaf. Gently brush egg mixture evenly over loaf. Bake 30 to 35 minutes or until loaf sounds hollow when tapped.

8. Remove immediately from cookie sheet. Cool completely on wire rack.   *Makes 12 servings*

Nutrients per Serving: 1 slice (1/12 of loaf)

Calories 124	**Fiber** 1g
Fat 1g (sat <1g)	**Cholesterol** 18mg
Protein 4g	**Sodium** 152mg
Carbohydrate 25g	

Exchanges: 1-1/2 starch

Tip

Temperature is an important factor when working with yeast. If the dissolving liquid is too cold, yeast action is retarded. Too much heat will kill the yeast. Use an instant-read thermometer to accurately determine if the liquid has reached the temperature called for in the recipe.

Soda Bread

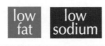 low fat | low sodium

- **1-1/2 cups whole wheat flour**
- **1 cup all-purpose flour**
- **1/2 cup rolled oats**
- **1/4 cup sugar**
- **1-1/2 teaspoons baking powder**
- **1/2 teaspoon baking soda**
- **1/4 teaspoon ground cinnamon**
- **1/3 cup raisins (optional)**
- **1/4 cup walnuts (optional)**
- **1-1/4 cups low-fat buttermilk**
- **1 tablespoon vegetable oil**

Preheat oven to 375°F. Combine flours, oats, sugar, baking powder, baking soda and cinnamon in large bowl. Stir in raisins and walnuts, if desired. Gradually stir in buttermilk and oil until dough forms. Knead in bowl 30 seconds. Spray 8×4-inch loaf pan with nonstick cooking spray; place dough in pan. Bake 40 to 50 minutes or until wooden pick inserted into center comes out clean. *Makes 16 slices*

Favorite recipe from **The Sugar Association, Inc.**

Nutrients per Serving: 1 slice (1/16 of loaf)

Calories 103	**Fiber** 2g
Fat 1g (sat <1g)	**Cholesterol** 1mg
Protein 3g	**Sodium** 77mg
Carbohydrate 20g	

Exchanges: 1-1/2 starch

Pull-Apart Rye Rolls

low fat

(Pictured at right)

- **3/4 cup water**
- **2 tablespoons margarine or butter, softened**
- **2 tablespoons molasses**
- **2-1/4 cups all-purpose flour, divided**
- **1/2 cup rye flour**
- **1/3 cup nonfat dry milk powder**
- **1 package (1/4 ounce) active dry yeast**
- **1-1/2 teaspoons salt**
- **1-1/2 teaspoons caraway seeds**
- **Melted margarine or vegetable oil**

1. Heat water, 2 tablespoons margarine and molasses in small saucepan over low heat until temperature reaches 120° to 130°F. Combine 1-1/4 cups all-purpose flour, rye flour, milk powder, yeast, salt and caraway seeds in large bowl. Stir heated water mixture into flour mixture with wooden spoon to form soft but sticky dough. Gradually add more all-purpose flour until rough dough forms.

2. Turn out dough onto lightly floured surface. Knead 5 to 8 minutes or until smooth and elastic, gradually adding remaining flour to prevent sticking, if necessary. Cover with inverted bowl. Let rise 35 to 40 minutes or until dough has increased in bulk by one third. Punch down dough; divide in half. Roll each half into 12-inch log. Using sharp knife, cut each log evenly into 12 pieces; shape into tight balls. Arrange in greased 8- or 9-inch cake pan. Brush tops with melted margarine. Loosely cover with lightly greased sheet of plastic wrap. Let rise in warm place 45 minutes or until doubled in bulk.

3. Preheat oven to 375°F. Uncover rolls; bake 15 to 20 minutes or until golden brown. Cool in pan on wire rack 5 minutes. Remove from pan. Cool completely on wire rack. *Makes 24 rolls*

Nutrients per Serving: 1 Roll

Calories 67	**Fiber** 1g
Fat 1g (sat <1g)	**Cholesterol** 3mg
Protein 2g	**Sodium** 150mg
Carbohydrate 12g	

Exchanges: 1 starch

Pull-Apart Rye Rolls

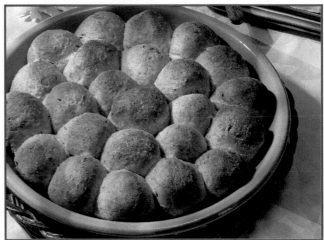

Blueberry-Sour Cream Corn Muffins

(Pictured at right)

    1 cup all-purpose flour
    3/4 cup cornmeal
    2 teaspoons baking powder
    1/2 teaspoon baking soda
    1/4 teaspoon salt
    1 egg, beaten
    1 cup reduced-fat sour cream
    1/3 cup thawed frozen unsweetened apple
        juice concentrate
    1-1/2 cups fresh or frozen (not thawed)
        blueberries
    2/3 cup reduced-fat whipped cream cheese
    2 tablespoons no-sugar-added blueberry
        fruit spread

1. Preheat oven to 400°F. Spray 12 medium-sized muffin cups with nonstick cooking spray, or line with paper liners; set aside.

2. Combine flour, cornmeal, baking powder, baking soda and salt in medium bowl. Add combined egg, sour cream and apple juice concentrate; mix just until dry ingredients are moistened. Gently stir in blueberries.

3. Spoon batter into prepared muffin cups, filling each cup 3/4 full. Bake 18 to 20 minutes or until golden brown. Let stand in pan on wire rack 5 minutes. Remove from pan; cool slightly. Combine cream cheese and fruit spread; serve with warm muffins.   *Makes 1 dozen muffins*

Nutrients per Serving: 1 Muffin with about 1 tablespoon spread

Calories 150	**Fiber** 1g
Fat 4g (sat 3g)	**Cholesterol** 29mg
Protein 5g	**Sodium** 252mg
Carbohydrate 23g	

Exchanges: 1 starch, 1/2 fruit, 1 fat

Banana Bran Loaf

    1 cup mashed ripe bananas (about
        2 large)
    1/2 cup granulated sugar
    1/3 cup (5-1/3 tablespoons) margarine or
        butter, melted
    1/3 cup fat-free milk
    2 egg whites, lightly beaten
    1-1/4 cups all-purpose flour
    1 cup QUAKER® Oat Bran hot cereal,
        uncooked
    2 teaspoons baking powder
    1/2 teaspoon baking soda

Heat oven to 350°F. Lightly spray 8×4-inch or 9×5-inch loaf pan with vegetable oil cooking spray or oil lightly. Combine bananas, sugar, melted margarine, milk and egg whites; mix well. Add combined flour, oat bran, baking powder and baking soda, mixing just until moistened. Pour into prepared pan. Bake 55 to 60 minutes or until wooden pick inserted into center comes out clean. Cool 10 minutes; remove from pan. Cool completely on wire rack.   *Makes 1 loaf (16 servings)*

Note: To freeze bread slices, layer waxed paper between each slice. Wrap bread securely in foil or place in freezer bag. Seal, label and freeze. To reheat, unwrap frozen bread slices and wrap in paper towel. Microwave at HIGH (100% power) about 30 seconds for each slice or until warm.

Nutrients per Serving: 1 slice (1/16 of loaf)

Calories 128	**Fiber** 2g
Fat 4g (sat <1g)	**Cholesterol** <1mg
Protein 3g	**Sodium** 155mg
Carbohydrate 20g	

Exchanges: 1 starch, 1 fat

Blueberry-Sour Cream Corn Muffins

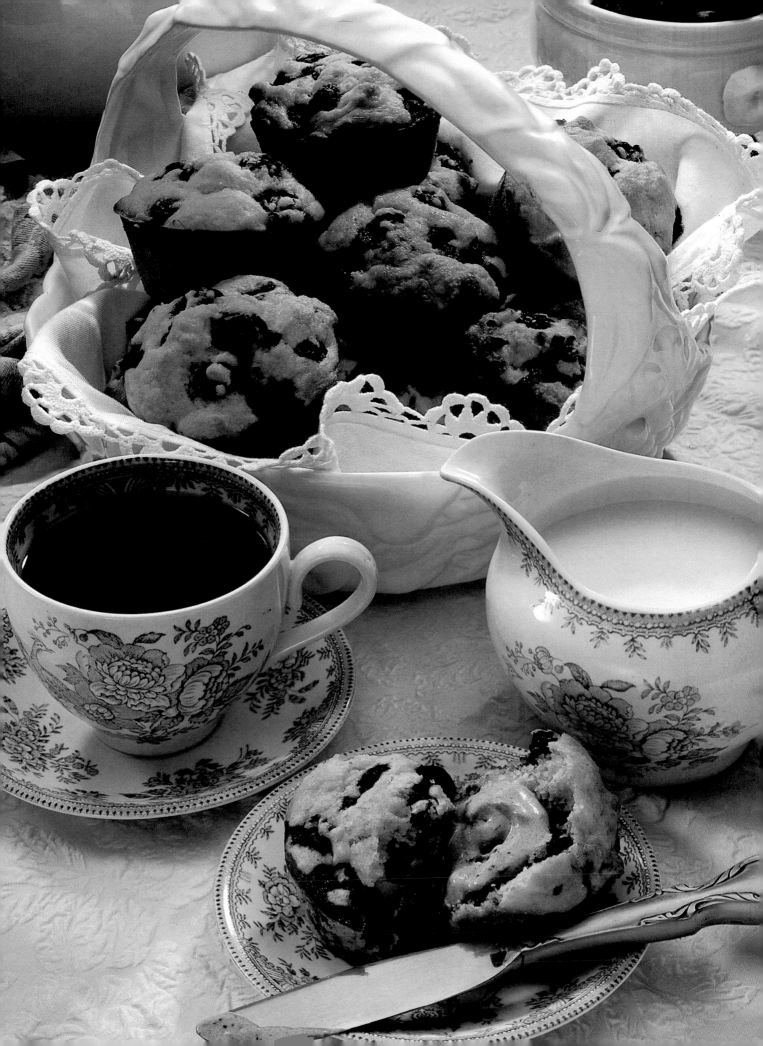

Greek Spinach-Cheese Rolls

low fat

(Pictured at right)

1 loaf (1 pound) frozen bread dough
1 package (10 ounces) frozen chopped
   spinach, thawed and squeezed dry
3/4 cup (3 ounces) crumbled feta cheese
1/2 cup (2 ounces) shredded reduced-fat
   Monterey Jack cheese
4 green onions, thinly sliced
1 teaspoon dried dill weed
1/2 teaspoon garlic powder
1/2 teaspoon black pepper

1. Thaw bread dough according to package directions. Spray 15 muffin cups with nonstick cooking spray; set aside. Roll out dough on lightly floured surface to 15×9-inch rectangle. (If dough is springy and difficult to roll, cover with plastic wrap and let rest 5 minutes to relax.) Position dough so long edge runs parallel to edge of work surface.

2. Combine spinach, cheeses, green onions, dill weed, garlic powder and pepper in large bowl; mix well. Sprinkle spinach mixture evenly over dough to within 1 inch of long edges. Starting at long edge, roll up snugly, pinching seam closed. Place seam-side down; cut roll with serrated knife into 1-inch-wide slices. Place slices, cut sides up, in prepared muffin cups. Cover with plastic wrap; let stand 30 minutes in warm place until rolls are slightly puffy.

3. Preheat oven to 375°F. Bake rolls 20 to 25 minutes or until golden. Serve warm or at room temperature. Rolls can be stored in refrigerator in airtight container up to 2 days. Garnish, if desired. *Makes 15 rolls*

Nutrients per Serving: 1 Roll

Calories 111	**Fiber** <1g
Fat 3g (sat 2g)	**Cholesterol** 8mg
Protein 5g	**Sodium** 267mg
Carbohydrate 16g	

Exchanges: 1 starch, 1/2 lean meat, 1/2 fat

Honey Wheat Bread

low fat

1-POUND LOAF
   3/4 cup plus 2 tablespoons water
   1-1/2 tablespoons margarine
   2 tablespoons honey
   1-1/2 cups bread flour
   1 cup whole wheat flour
   1 tablespoon brown sugar
   1 tablespoon nonfat dry milk
   1 teaspoon salt
   1-1/2 teaspoons active dry yeast

1-1/2-POUND LOAF
   1-1/4 cups water
   2 tablespoons margarine
   3 tablespoons honey
   2 cups bread flour
   1-1/2 cups whole wheat flour
   2 tablespoons brown sugar
   2 tablespoons nonfat dry milk
   1-1/2 teaspoons salt
   2 teaspoons active dry yeast

1. Measuring carefully, place all ingredients in bread machine pan in order specified by owner's manual.

2. Program desired cycle and crust setting; press start. Remove baked bread from pan; cool on wire rack. *Makes 1 loaf*

Favorite recipe from **North Dakota Wheat Commission**

Nutrients per Serving: 1 slice (1/12 of 1-pound loaf)

Calories 126	**Fiber** 2g
Fat 2g (sat <1g)	**Cholesterol** <1mg
Protein 4g	**Sodium** 214mg
Carbohydrate 24g	

Exchanges: 1-1/2 starch

Greek Spinach-Cheese Rolls

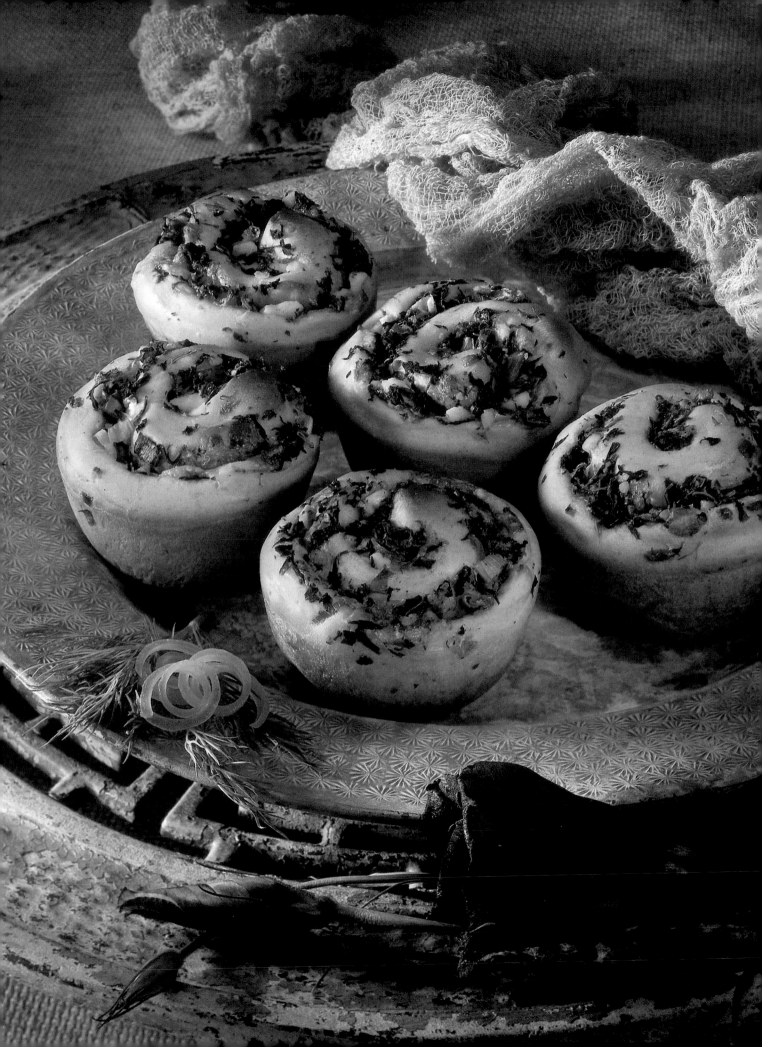

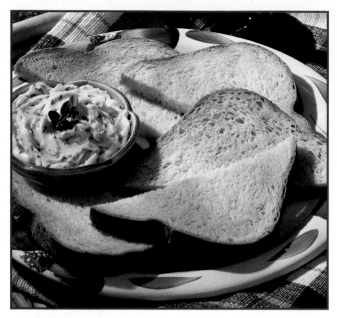

Potato Bread

Potato Bread

low fat

(Pictured above)

1-1/2-POUND LOAF
1-1/3 cups water
1-1/2 tablespoons margarine or butter
1-1/2 teaspoons salt
   3 cups bread flour
  1/2 cup mashed potato flakes
    2 tablespoons sugar
    2 tablespoons nonfat dry milk powder
1-1/2 teaspoons rapid-rise active dry yeast

2-POUND LOAF
1-3/4 cups water
   2 tablespoons margarine or butter
   2 teaspoons salt
   4 cups bread flour
  3/4 cup mashed potato flakes
   3 tablespoons sugar
   3 tablespoons nonfat dry milk powder
   2 teaspoons rapid-rise active dry yeast

1. Measuring carefully, place all ingredients in bread machine pan in order specified by owner's manual.

2. Program basic cycle and desired crust setting; press start. Remove baked bread from pan; cool on wire rack. *Makes 12 servings*

50 *Breads*

əə əə əə

Blueberry-Orange Bread

low fat

    1 cup FIBER ONE® cereal
  3/4 cup water
  1/4 cup orange juice
    1 tablespoon grated orange or lemon peel
  1/2 teaspoon vanilla
    2 cups GOLD MEDAL® all-purpose flour
    1 cup sugar
1-1/2 teaspoons baking powder
  1/2 teaspoon baking soda
  1/2 teaspoon salt
    2 tablespoons vegetable oil
    1 egg
    1 cup fresh or thawed frozen blueberries

1. Heat oven to 350°F. Grease bottom only of 9×5×3-inch loaf pan.

2. Crush cereal.* Stir together cereal, water, orange juice, orange peel and vanilla in large bowl; let stand 10 minutes. Stir in remaining ingredients except blueberries. Gently stir in blueberries. Pour into pan.

3. Bake 50 to 60 minutes or until toothpick inserted into center comes out clean. Cool 10 minutes. Loosen sides of loaf; remove from pan. Cool completely before slicing.
Makes 1 loaf (24 slices)

*Place cereal in plastic bag or between sheets of waxed paper and crush with rolling pin.

Pan de Pueblo

1-1/4 cups warm water (100° to 110°F)
1 envelope FLEISCHMANN'S® Active Dry Yeast
2 teaspoons coarse salt
3-1/4 cups all-purpose flour
Cornmeal

EGG WHITE MIXTURE
1 egg white, lightly beaten with
1 teaspoon water

Place 1/4 cup warm water in large warm bowl. Sprinkle in yeast; stir until dissolved. Add remaining water, salt and 1 cup flour. Beat 2 minutes at medium speed of electric mixer, scraping bowl occasionally. Add 1/2 cup flour; beat 2 minutes at high speed. Stir in enough remaining flour to make a soft dough. Knead on lightly floured surface until smooth and elastic, about 8 to 10 minutes. Place in bowl coated with nonstick cooking spray, turning to coat top. Cover; let rise in warm, draft-free place until doubled in size, about 1-1/2 hours.

Punch dough down. Remove dough to lightly floured surface; divide into 2 equal portions. Roll each piece into 20×5-inch oblong. Starting with long side, roll up tightly as for jelly-roll. Pinch seam and ends to seal. Place seam side down and diagonally on a baking sheet that has been sprinkled with cornmeal. Slit the tops several times diagonally with a sharp knife. Cover; let rise in warm, draft-free place until doubled in size, about 1 hour.

Bake at 450°F for 5 minutes with a pan of water on the oven floor. Remove the pan of water and continue baking the bread 5 minutes more. Brush bread with egg white mixture. Bake an additional 5 to 10 minutes or until brown and crusty. Remove from sheets; cool on wire racks.

Makes 2 loaves

Nutrients per Serving: 1 slice (1/12 of 1 loaf)

Calories 70	**Fiber** <1g
Fat 0g (sat 0g)	**Cholesterol** 0mg
Protein 2g	**Sodium** 200mg
Carbohydrate 14g	

Exchanges: 1 starch

Cornmeal Scones

(Pictured on page 32)

1/2 cup dried currants
1 cup warm water
1-1/3 cups all-purpose flour
2/3 cup cornmeal
1/2 cup plus 1 teaspoon sugar, divided
1-1/2 teaspoons baking powder
1/2 teaspoon baking soda
1/4 teaspoon salt
1/4 cup cold margarine, cut into 4 pieces
1/4 cup plain fat-free yogurt
3 tablespoons fat-free milk
1 egg, lightly beaten
1 egg white, lightly beaten

1. Preheat oven to 375°F. Lightly spray baking sheet with nonstick cooking spray; set aside.

2. Place currants in small mixing bowl. Add water. Let stand 10 minutes; drain and discard water.

3. Combine flour, cornmeal, 1/2 cup sugar, baking powder, baking soda and salt in large mixing bowl. Cut margarine into flour mixture with pastry blender or 2 knives until mixture resembles coarse crumbs. Stir in currants.

4. Combine yogurt, milk and egg in small bowl. Add to flour mixture, stirring just until dry ingredients are moistened.

5. Turn out dough onto lightly floured surface; knead 5 or 6 times. Shape dough into 8-inch round. Place on baking sheet. Brush with egg white; sprinkle with remaining 1 teaspoon sugar. Cut into 8 wedges. Bake 20 minutes or until lightly browned. Place on wire rack to cool. Cut each wedge in half to make 16 servings.

Makes 16 servings

Nutrients per Serving: 1 Scone

Calories 132	**Fiber** 1g
Fat 3g (sat 1g)	**Cholesterol** 13mg
Protein 3g	**Sodium** 170mg
Carbohydrate 22g	

Exchanges: 1-1/2 starch, 1/2 fat

Red Pepper Bread

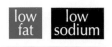

(Pictured at right)

2 to 2-1/2 cups all-purpose flour, divided
1 cup whole wheat flour
2 tablespoons grated Parmesan cheese
1 teaspoon dried rosemary leaves
1 package rapid-rise active dry yeast
1/2 teaspoon salt
1/4 teaspoon dried thyme leaves
1-1/4 cups hot water (130°F)
1 tablespoon olive or vegetable oil
1/2 cup chopped roasted red pepper
1 egg white, beaten
2 teaspoons water
Additional dried rosemary leaves
(optional)

1. Combine 1 cup all-purpose flour, whole wheat flour, cheese, 1 teaspoon rosemary, yeast, salt and thyme in large bowl. Stir in hot water and oil until mixture is smooth; stir in red pepper. Stir in enough remaining all-purpose flour to form soft dough. Turn dough out onto lightly floured surface; flatten slightly. Knead gently 2 to 3 minutes or until smooth and elastic, adding additional all-purpose flour to prevent sticking, if necessary. Place dough in large bowl sprayed with nonstick cooking spray. Turn dough over to coat top with cooking spray. Let rise, covered, in warm place 30 minutes or until doubled in bulk. Punch down dough.

2. Shape dough into 1 large or 2 small round or long loaves on cookie sheet coated with nonstick cooking spray. Let stand, covered, 30 minutes or until doubled in bulk.

3. Preheat oven to 375°F. Slash top of dough with sharp knife. Mix egg white and 2 teaspoons water in small cup; brush over dough and sprinkle with additional rosemary, if desired.

4. Bake 35 to 40 minutes for 1 large loaf, 25 to 30 minutes for 2 small loaves or until bread is golden and sounds hollow when gently tapped. Cool on wire rack.

Makes 20 slices (1 large loaf or
2 small loaves)

Nutrients per Serving: 1 slice (1/20 of 1 large loaf)

Calories 78	**Fiber** 1g
Fat 1g (sat <1g)	**Cholesterol** <1mg
Protein 3g	**Sodium** 80mg
Carbohydrate 14g	

Exchanges: 1 starch

❧ ❧ ❧

Super Brown Bread

2 cups warm water (105° to 115°F)
2 packages active dry yeast
1-1/2 cups whole wheat flour
2-1/2 to 3 cups bread flour, divided
1/2 cup rolled oats
1/2 cup packed brown sugar
1/4 cup wheat germ
1/4 cup vegetable oil
1/4 cup molasses
2 teaspoons salt

In large bowl, combine water and yeast. Let stand until dissolved, about 5 minutes. Add whole wheat flour, 1 cup bread flour, oats, brown sugar, wheat germ, oil, molasses and salt. Beat until smooth. Add additional bread flour to make soft dough.

Knead 10 minutes or until smooth. Place in greased bowl, turning to grease top; cover and let rise until doubled.

Form into two loaves; place in two 8×4-inch greased loaf pans and let rise until doubled. Bake at 450°F for 10 minutes. *Reduce oven temperature to 325°F; bake 35 minutes.*

Makes 2 loaves (16 slices each)

Favorite recipe from **North Dakota Wheat Commission**

Nutrients per Serving: 1 slice (1/16 of 1 loaf)

Calories 103	**Fiber** 1g
Fat 2g (sat <1g)	**Cholesterol** 0mg
Protein 3g	**Sodium** 148mg
Carbohydrate 19g	

Exchanges: 1 starch, 1/2 fat

Red Pepper Bread

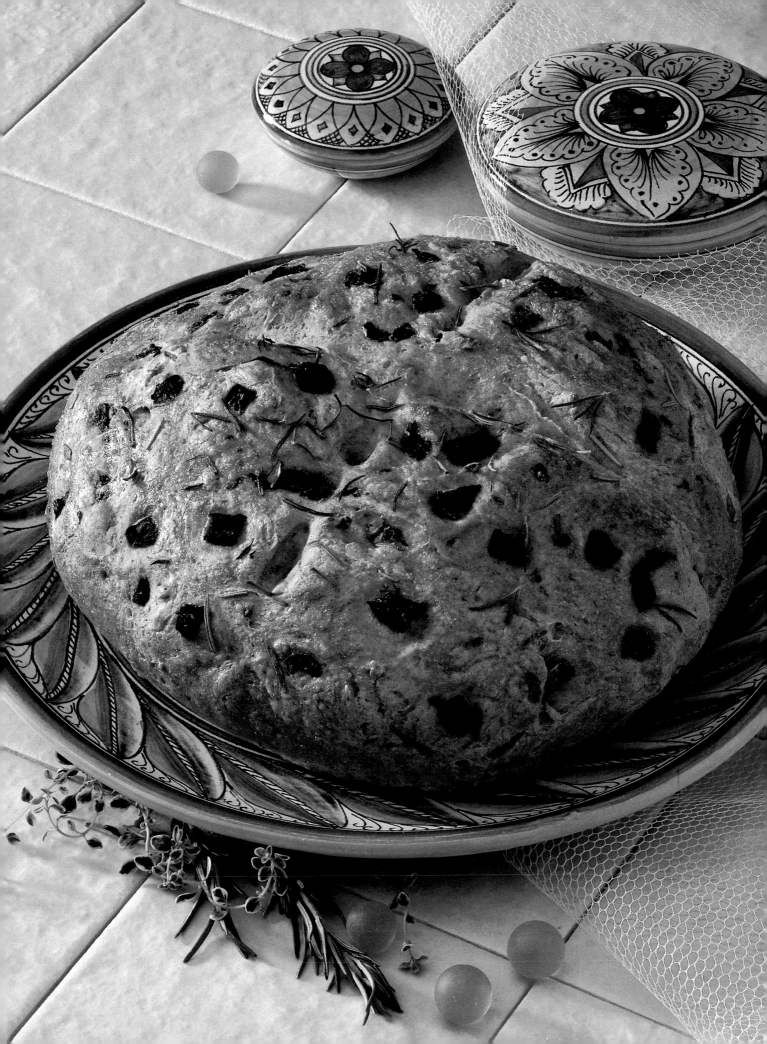

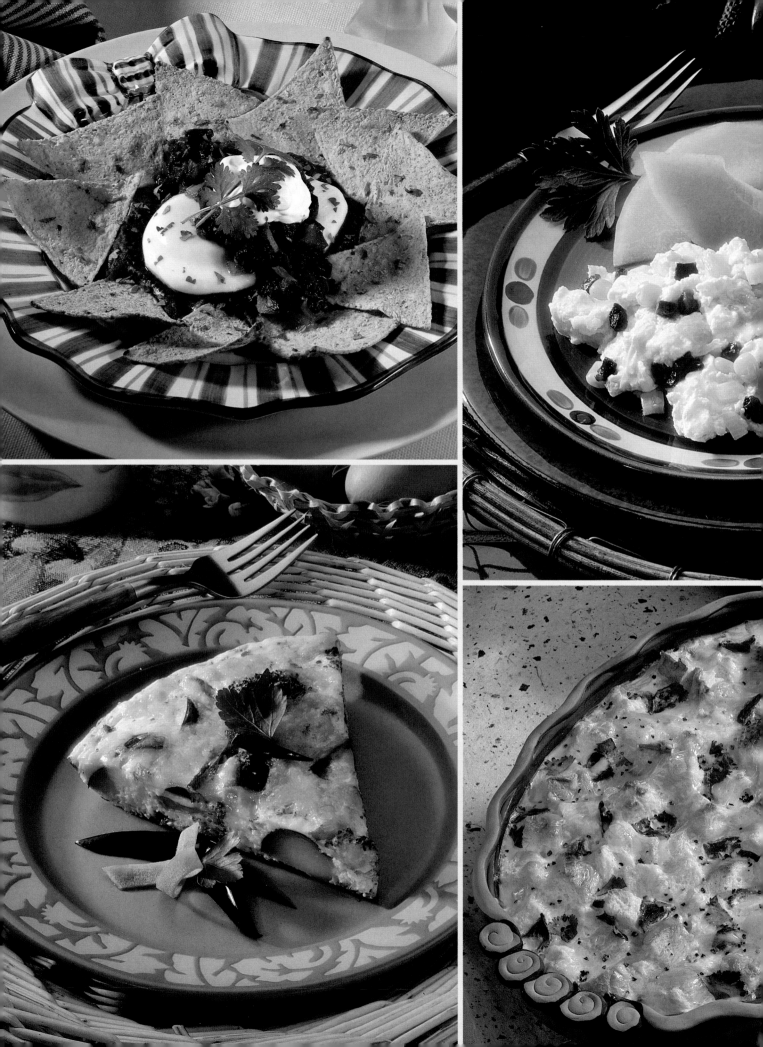

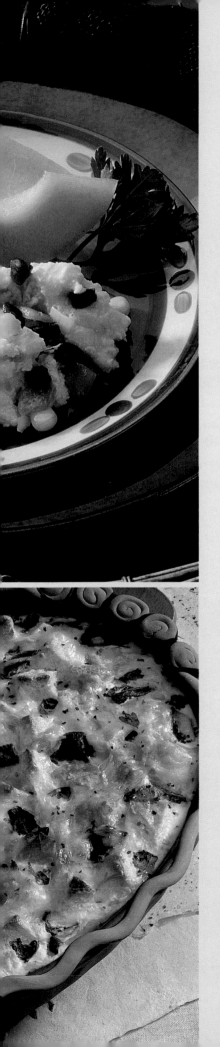

Breakfast & Brunch

ঙ ঙ ঙ

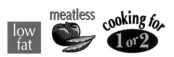

Chile Scramble

Quick Recipe   *(Pictured at left)*

> **2 tablespoons minced onion**
> **1 teaspoon FLEISCHMANN'S® Original Margarine**
> **1 cup EGG BEATERS® Healthy Real Egg Product**
> **1 (4-ounce) can diced green chiles, drained**
> **1/4 cup whole kernel corn**
> **2 tablespoons diced pimientos**

In 10-inch nonstick skillet, over medium-high heat, sauté onion in margarine for 2 to 3 minutes or until onion is translucent.

Pour Egg Beaters® into skillet; cook, stirring occasionally, until mixture is set.

Stir in chiles, corn and pimientos; cook 1 minute more or until heated through.   *Makes 2 servings*

Nutrients per Serving: 1/2 of total recipe

Calories 122	**Fiber** 3g
Fat 2g (sat <1g)	**Cholesterol** 0mg
Protein 13g	**Sodium** 427mg
Carbohydrate 13g	

Exchanges: 2 vegetable, 1-1/2 lean meat

Clockwise from top left: *Eggs Santa Fe (page 60), Chile Scramble, Roasted Pepper and Sourdough Brunch Casserole (page 63) and Farmstand Frittata (page 58)*

Triple-Decker Vegetable Omelet

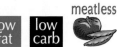 low fat | low carb | meatless

Quick Recipe (Pictured at right)

    1 cup finely chopped broccoli
1/2 cup diced red bell pepper
1/2 cup shredded carrot
1/3 cup sliced green onions
    1 clove garlic, minced
2-1/2 teaspoons FLEISCHMANN'S® Original
         Margarine, divided
3/4 cup low fat cottage cheese (1% milkfat),
         divided
    1 tablespoon plain dry bread crumbs
    1 tablespoon grated Parmesan cheese
1/2 teaspoon Italian seasoning
1-1/2 cups EGG BEATERS® Healthy Real Egg
         Product, divided
1/3 cup chopped tomato
    Chopped fresh parsley, for garnish

In 8-inch nonstick skillet, over medium-high heat, sauté broccoli, bell pepper, carrot, green onions and garlic in 1 teaspoon margarine until tender. Remove from skillet; stir in 1/2 cup cottage cheese. Keep warm. Combine bread crumbs, Parmesan cheese and Italian seasoning; set aside.

In same skillet, over medium heat, melt 1/2 teaspoon margarine. Pour 1/2 cup Egg Beaters® into skillet. Cook, lifting edges to allow uncooked portion to flow underneath. When almost set, slide unfolded omelet onto ovenproof serving platter. Top with half each of the vegetable mixture and bread crumb mixture; set aside.

Prepare 2 more omelets with remaining Egg Beaters® and margarine. Layer 1 omelet onto serving platter over vegetable and bread crumb mixture; top with remaining vegetable mixture and bread crumb mixture. Layer with remaining omelet. Top omelet with remaining cottage cheese and tomato. Bake at 425°F for 5 to 7 minutes or until heated through. Garnish with parsley. Cut into wedges to serve.

Makes 4 servings

Nutrients per Serving: 1 wedge (1/4 of total recipe)

Calories 130	**Fiber** 2g
Fat 3g (sat 1g)	**Cholesterol** 3mg
Protein 16g	**Sodium** 411mg
Carbohydrate 9g	

Exchanges: 1 vegetable, 2 lean meat

⁓ ⁓ ⁓

Peaches and Creamy Dip with Waffle Wedges

low fat | low sodium

Quick Recipe

    4 ounces reduced-fat cream cheese
1/3 cup no-sugar-added peach preserves
    1 tablespoon fat-free milk
    2 packages sugar substitute*
1/2 teaspoon vanilla extract
    4 low-fat toaster waffles
    Ground cinnamon to taste

*This recipe was tested with Equal® sweetener.

1. Place all ingredients except waffles and cinnamon in blender and process until smooth. Set aside.

2. Toast waffles and cut each waffle into 6 wedges.

3. Place cream cheese mixture in small serving bowl and sprinkle with cinnamon. Serve with waffle wedges for dipping.

Makes 24 servings (24 wedges and about 3/4 cup dip)

Nutrients per Serving: 1 Wedge with about 1-1/2 teaspoons Dip

Calories 54	**Fiber** <1g
Fat 3g (sat <1g)	**Cholesterol** <1mg
Protein 2g	**Sodium** 57mg
Carbohydrate 5g	

Exchanges: 1/2 starch

Triple-Decker Vegetable Omelet

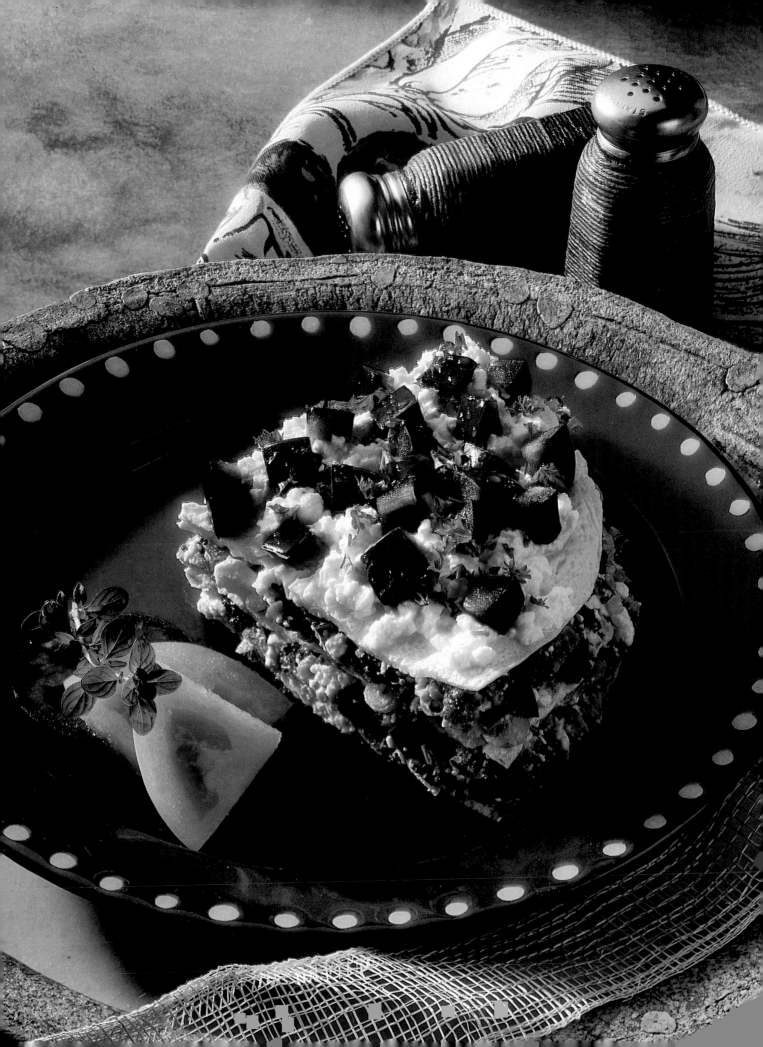

Apricot Walnut Swirl Coffee Cake

WALNUT FILLING

   1/2 cup sugar-free apricot preserves or apricot spreadable fruit

   3/4 cup EQUAL® SPOONFUL*

   4 teaspoons ground cinnamon

   1/2 cup chopped walnuts

COFFEE CAKE

   2-1/3 cups reduced-fat baking mix (Bisquick®)

   1/2 cup EQUAL® SPOONFUL**

   2/3 cup fat-free milk

   1/3 cup fat-free sour cream

   1 egg

   2 tablespoons stick butter or margarine, melted

   1/3 cup sugar-free apricot preserves or apricot spreadable fruit

May substitute 18 packets Equal® sweetener.

**May substitute 12 packets Equal® sweetener.*

• For Walnut Filling, mix 1/2 cup apricot preserves, 3/4 cup Equal® Spoonful, cinnamon and walnuts in small bowl.

• For Coffee Cake, combine baking mix and 1/2 cup Equal® Spoonful; mix in milk, sour cream, egg and butter. Spread 1/3 of batter in greased and floured 6-cup bundt pan; spoon half of Walnut Filling over batter. Repeat layers, ending with batter.

• Bake in preheated 375°F oven about 25 minutes or until coffee cake is browned on top and toothpick inserted into center comes out clean. Cool in pan 5 minutes; invert onto wire rack and cool 5 to 10 minutes.

• Spoon 1/3 cup apricot preserves over top of coffee cake; serve warm.　*Makes 12 servings*

Nutrients per Serving: 1 slice (1/12 of Coffee Cake)

Calories 189	**Fiber** 1g
Fat 7g (sat 1g)	**Cholesterol** 18mg
Protein 4g	**Sodium** 332mg
Carbohydrate 28g	

Exchanges: 2 starch, 1 fat

Farmstand Frittata

(Pictured on page 54)

   Nonstick cooking spray

   1/2 cup chopped onion

   1 medium red bell pepper, seeded and cut into thin strips

   1 cup broccoli florets, blanched and drained

   1 cup cooked, quartered, unpeeled red potatoes

   1 cup cholesterol-free egg substitute

   6 egg whites

   1 tablespoon chopped fresh parsley

   1/2 teaspoon salt

   1/4 teaspoon black pepper

   1/2 cup (2 ounces) shredded reduced-fat Cheddar cheese

1. Spray large nonstick ovenproof skillet with cooking spray; heat over medium heat until hot. Add onion and bell pepper; cook and stir 3 minutes or until crisp-tender.

2. Add broccoli and potatoes; cook and stir 1 to 2 minutes or until heated through.

3. Whisk together egg substitute, egg whites, parsley, salt and black pepper in medium bowl.

4. Spread vegetables into even layer in skillet. Pour egg white mixture over vegetables; cover and cook over medium heat 10 to 12 minutes or until egg mixture is set.

5. Meanwhile, preheat broiler. Top frittata with cheese. Broil 4 inches from heat 1 minute or until cheese is bubbly and golden brown. Cut into 4 wedges. Garnish, if desired.

Makes 4 servings

Nutrients per Serving: 1 Frittata wedge (1/4 of total recipe)

Calories 163	**Fiber** 2g
Fat 2g (sat 1g)	**Cholesterol** 8mg
Protein 17g	**Sodium** 686mg
Carbohydrate 19g	

Exchanges: 1 starch, 2 lean meat

Brunch Strata

(Pictured below right)

1 can (10-3/4 ounces) reduced-fat condensed cream of celery soup, undiluted

2 cups cholesterol-free egg substitute or 8 eggs

1 cup fat-free milk

1 can (4 ounces) sliced mushrooms

1/4 cup sliced green onions

1 teaspoon dry mustard

1/2 teaspoon salt (optional)

1/4 teaspoon black pepper

6 slices reduced-fat white bread, cut into 1-inch cubes

4 links reduced-fat precooked breakfast sausage, thinly sliced

1. Preheat oven to 350°F. Spray 2-quart baking dish with nonstick cooking spray; set aside.

2. Combine soup, egg substitute, milk, mushrooms, green onions, mustard, salt, if desired, and pepper in medium bowl; mix well.

3. Combine bread cubes, sausage and soup mixture in prepared baking dish; toss to coat. Bake 30 to 35 minutes or until set. Garnish as desired.   *Makes 6 servings*

Nutrients per Serving: 1 cup Strata

Calories 155	**Fiber** 3g
Fat 2g (sat 1g)	**Cholesterol** 8mg
Protein 15g	**Sodium** 642mg
Carbohydrate 20g	

Exchanges: 1 starch, 2 lean meat

Tip

By using egg substitute instead of the whole eggs in this recipe, you are reducing the amount of fat by nearly 5 grams per serving and the amount of cholesterol by nearly 212 milligrams per serving!

Fitness Shake

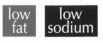

Quick Recipe

2 cups skim milk

2 medium-size ripe bananas, cut into 1-inch pieces

1/2 cup plain or banana nonfat yogurt

1/2 cup nonfat dry milk powder

1/3 cup wheat germ

1 teaspoon vanilla

2-1/2 teaspoons EQUAL® FOR RECIPES or 8 packets EQUAL® sweetener or 1/3 cup EQUAL® SPOONFUL™

Ground cinnamon (optional)

• Blend all ingredients except cinnamon in blender or food processor until smooth. Pour into glasses and sprinkle with cinnamon, if desired.   *Makes 4 (8-ounce) servings*

Nutrients per Serving: 1 Shake (8 ounces)

Calories 190	**Fiber** 3g
Fat 2g (sat <1g)	**Cholesterol** 5mg
Protein 12g	**Sodium** 137mg
Carbohydrate 34g	

Exchanges: 1/2 starch, 1 fruit, 1 milk

Brunch Strata

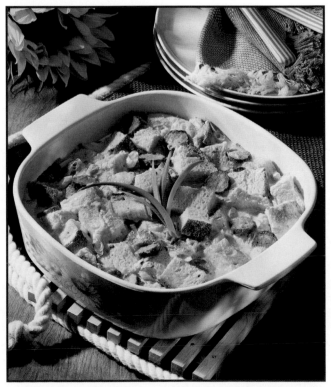

Spinach Feta Frittata

Quick Recipe   *(Pictured at right)*

1-1/2 cups cholesterol-free egg substitute

1/3 cup evaporated fat-free milk

1 package (10-ounces) frozen chopped spinach, thawed and squeezed dry

1/2 cup finely chopped green onions

1-1/2 teaspoons dried oregano or basil leaves

1/4 teaspoon salt

1/8 teaspoon black pepper

2 cups cooked spaghetti noodles (4 ounces uncooked)

1 cup (4 ounces) crumbled sun-dried tomato and basil or plain feta

Nonstick cooking spray

Diced red bell pepper (optional)

1. Preheat broiler.

2. Combine egg substitute and milk in medium bowl; whisk together until well blended. Stir in spinach, green onions, oregano, salt and black pepper. Stir in noodles and feta.

3. Spray 10-inch cast iron or ovenproof skillet with cooking spray. Heat over medium heat. Add egg mixture and cook 5 minutes or until nearly cooked through, stirring occasionally.

4. Place skillet under broiler 3 to 5 minutes or until just beginning to lightly brown and set.

5. Remove from broiler. Cut into 4 wedges. Top each wedge with diced bell pepper, if desired.

Makes 4 servings

Nutrients per Serving: 1 Frittata wedge

Calories 254	**Fiber** 4g
Fat 7g (sat 5g)	**Cholesterol** 21mg
Protein 20g	**Sodium** 762mg
Carbohydrate 26g	

Exchanges: 1 starch, 2 vegetable, 2-1/2 lean meat

Eggs Santa Fe

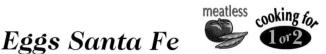

Quick Recipe   *(Pictured on page 54)*

2 eggs

1/2 cup GUILTLESS GOURMET® Black Bean Dip (Spicy or Mild)

1/4 cup GUILTLESS GOURMET® Southwestern Grill Salsa

1 ounce (about 20) GUILTLESS GOURMET® Unsalted Baked Tortilla Chips

2 tablespoons low fat sour cream

1 teaspoon chopped fresh cilantro

Fresh cilantro sprigs (optional)

To poach eggs, bring water to a boil in small skillet over high heat; reduce heat to medium-low and maintain a simmer. Gently break eggs into water, being careful not to break yolks. Cover and simmer 5 minutes or until desired firmness.

Meanwhile, place bean dip in small microwave-safe bowl or small saucepan. Microwave bean dip on HIGH (100% power) 2 to 3 minutes or heat over medium heat until warm. To serve, spread 1/4 cup warm bean dip in center of serving plate; top with 1 poached egg and 2 tablespoons salsa. Arrange 10 tortilla chips around egg. Dollop with 1 tablespoon sour cream and sprinkle with 1/2 teaspoon chopped cilantro. Repeat with remaining ingredients. Garnish with cilantro sprigs, if desired.

Makes 2 servings

Nutrients per Serving: 1/2 of total recipe

Calories 220	**Fiber** 3g
Fat 7g (sat 3g)	**Cholesterol** 217mg
Protein 13g	**Sodium** 423mg
Carbohydrate 26g	

Exchanges: 2 starch, 1 lean meat, 1/2 fat

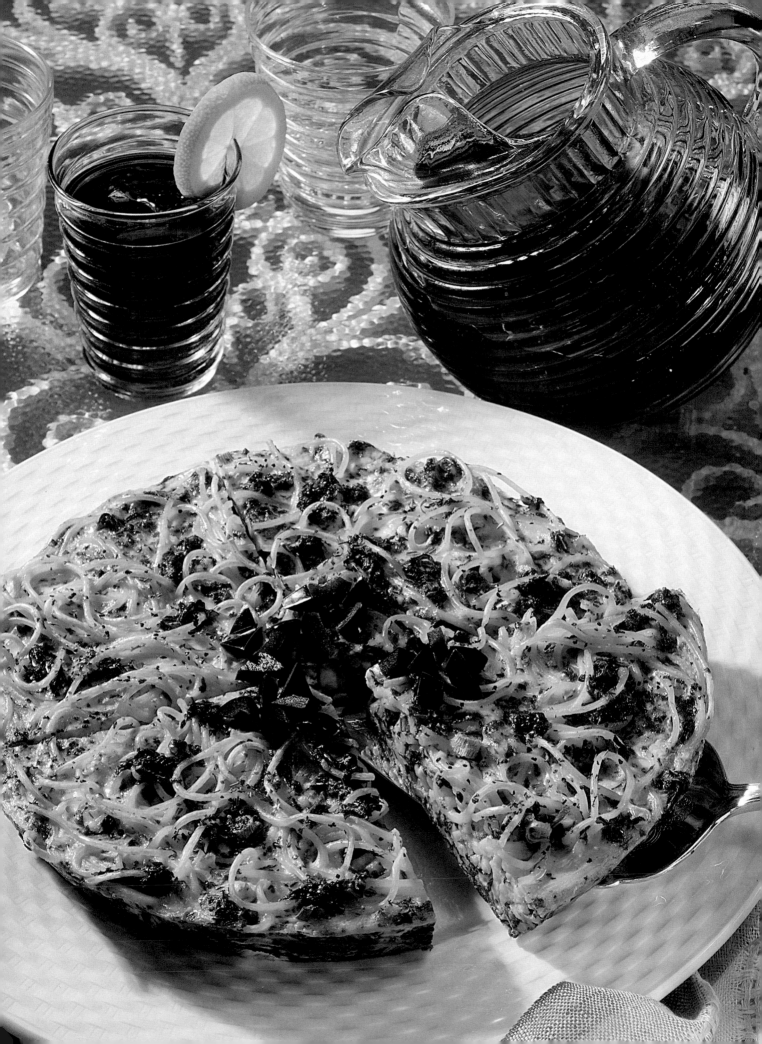

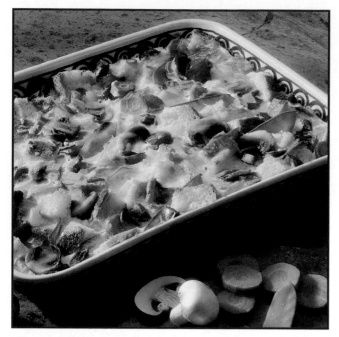

Vegetable Strata

and milk; pour over vegetable mixture. Bake at 375°F for 45 to 50 minutes or until knife inserted into center comes out clean. Let stand 10 minutes before serving.

Makes 6 servings

Nutrients per Serving: 1/6 of total recipe

Calories 83	**Fiber** 1g
Fat 1g (sat <1g)	**Cholesterol** 3mg
Protein 8g	**Sodium** 161mg
Carbohydrate 10g	

Exchanges: 2 vegetable, 1/2 lean meat

ɝ ɝ ɝ

Vegetable Strata

 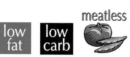

(Pictured above)

2 slices white bread, cubed
1/4 cup shredded reduced-fat Swiss cheese
1/2 cup sliced carrots
1/2 cup sliced mushrooms
1/4 cup chopped onion
1 clove garlic, crushed
1 teaspoon FLEISCHMANN'S® Original Margarine
1/2 cup chopped tomato
1/2 cup snow peas
1 cup EGG BEATERS® Healthy Real Egg Product
3/4 cup skim milk

Place bread cubes evenly on bottom of greased 1-1/2-quart casserole dish. Sprinkle with cheese; set aside.

In medium nonstick skillet, over medium heat, sauté carrots, mushrooms, onion and garlic in margarine until tender. Stir in tomato and snow peas; cook 1 to 2 minutes more. Spoon over cheese. In small bowl, combine Egg Beaters®

Mushroom-Herb Omelet

Quick Recipe

1 cup EGG BEATERS® Healthy Real Egg Product
1 tablespoon chopped fresh parsley
1 teaspoon finely chopped fresh oregano, basil or thyme (*or* 1/4 teaspoon dried)
2 cups sliced fresh mushrooms
2 teaspoons FLEISCHMANN'S® Original Margarine, divided

In small bowl, combine Egg Beaters®, parsley and oregano, basil or thyme; set aside.

In 8-inch nonstick skillet, over medium heat, sauté mushrooms in 1 teaspoon margarine until tender; set aside. In same skillet, over medium heat, melt 1/2 teaspoon margarine. Pour half the egg mixture into skillet. Cook, lifting edges to allow uncooked portion to flow underneath. When almost set, spoon half of mushrooms over half of omelet. Fold other half over mushrooms; slide onto serving plate. Repeat with remaining margarine, egg mixture and mushrooms.

Makes 2 servings

Nutrients per Serving: 1 Omelet (1/2 of total recipe)

Calories 114	**Fiber** 1g
Fat 3g (sat 1g)	**Cholesterol** 0mg
Protein 14g	**Sodium** 239mg
Carbohydrate 7g	

Exchanges: 1 vegetable, 2 lean meat

Banana Coffee Cake

1/2 cup 100% bran cereal
1/2 cup strong coffee
1 cup mashed ripe bananas
1/2 cup sugar
1 egg, lightly beaten
2 tablespoons canola oil
1/2 cup all-purpose flour
1/2 cup whole wheat flour
2 teaspoons baking powder
1 teaspoon ground cinnamon
1/4 teaspoon salt

1. Preheat oven to 350°F. Coat 8-inch square baking dish with nonstick cooking spray; set aside.

2. Combine bran cereal and coffee in large bowl; let stand 3 minutes or until cereal softens. Stir in bananas, sugar, egg and oil.

3. Combine all-purpose flour, whole wheat flour, baking powder, cinnamon and salt in small bowl; stir into banana mixture just until moistened. Pour into prepared dish.

4. Bake 25 to 35 minutes or until wooden toothpick inserted into center of cake comes out clean. Cool in dish on wire rack. Cut into 9 squares before serving.   *Makes 9 servings*

Nutrients per Serving: 1 Coffee Cake square (1/9 of total recipe)

Calories 169	**Fiber** 3g
Fat 4g (sat <1g)	**Cholesterol** 24mg
Protein 3g	**Sodium** 166mg
Carbohydrate 30g	

Exchanges: 1 starch, 1 fruit, 1 fat

Tip
About 2 large bananas yield 1 cup mashed bananas.

Roasted Pepper and Sourdough Brunch Casserole

meatless

(Pictured on page 54)

3 cups sourdough bread cubes
1 jar (12 ounces) roasted pepper strips, drained
1 cup (4 ounces) shredded reduced-fat sharp Cheddar cheese
1 cup (4 ounces) shredded reduced-fat Monterey Jack cheese
1 cup fat-free cottage cheese
12 ounces cholesterol-free egg substitute
1 cup fat-free milk
1/4 cup chopped fresh cilantro
1/4 teaspoon black pepper

1. Spray 11×7-inch baking pan with nonstick cooking spray. Place bread cubes in pan. Arrange roasted peppers evenly over bread cubes. Sprinkle Cheddar and Monterey Jack cheeses over peppers.

2. Place cottage cheese in food processor or blender; process until smooth. Add egg substitute; process 10 seconds.

3. Combine cottage cheese mixture and milk in small bowl; pour over ingredients in baking pan. Sprinkle with cilantro and black pepper. Cover with plastic wrap; refrigerate 4 to 12 hours.

4. Preheat oven to 375°F. Bake, uncovered, 40 minutes or until hot and bubbly and golden brown on top.   *Makes 8 servings*

Nutrients per Serving: about 3/4 cup Casserole

Calories 179	**Fiber** 1g
Fat 6g (sat 3g)	**Cholesterol** 22mg
Protein 19g	**Sodium** 704mg
Carbohydrate 13g	

Exchanges: 1 starch, 2 lean meat

Eggs Primavera

meatless

Quick Recipe   *(Pictured at right)*

**4 small round loaves (4 inches each)
whole wheat bread**
1-1/2 cups chopped onions
3/4 cup chopped yellow summer squash
3/4 cup chopped zucchini
1/2 cup chopped red bell pepper
**2 ounces snow peas, trimmed and cut
diagonally into thirds**
1/4 cup finely chopped fresh parsley
**1-1/2 teaspoons finely chopped fresh thyme
or 3/4 teaspoon dried thyme leaves**
**1 teaspoon finely chopped fresh rosemary
or 1/2 teaspoon dried rosemary
leaves, crushed**
2 whole eggs
4 egg whites
1/4 teaspoon black pepper
**1/2 cup (2 ounces) shredded reduced-fat
Swiss cheese**

1. Preheat oven to 350°F.

2. Slice top off each loaf of bread. Carefully hollow out each loaf, leaving sides and bottom 1/2 inch thick. Reserve centers for another use. Place loaves and tops, cut sides up, on baking sheet. Spray all surfaces with nonstick cooking spray; bake 15 minutes or until well toasted.

3. Spray large nonstick skillet with cooking spray and heat over medium heat until hot. Add onions; cook and stir 3 minutes or until soft. Add yellow squash, zucchini and bell pepper; cook and stir 3 minutes or until crisp-tender. Add snow peas and herbs; cook and stir 1 minute.

4. Whisk eggs, egg whites and black pepper in small bowl until blended. Add to vegetable mixture; gently stir until eggs begin to set. Sprinkle cheese over top; gently stir until cheese melts and eggs are set but not dry.

5. Fill each bread bowl with 1/4 of egg mixture, about 1 cup. Place tops back on bread bowls before serving. Garnish, if desired.

Makes 4 servings

Nutrients per Serving: 1 bread bowl filled with about 1 cup Egg mixture (1/4 of total recipe)

Calories 201	**Fiber** 4g
Fat 6g (sat 2g)	**Cholesterol** 114mg
Protein 14g	**Sodium** 336mg
Carbohydrate 23g	

Exchanges: 1 starch, 1 vegetable, 1-1/2 lean meat, 1/2 fat

❧ ❧ ❧

French Toast Sticks

meatless

Quick Recipe

**1 cup EGG BEATERS® Healthy Real Egg
Product**
1/3 cup skim milk
1 teaspoon ground cinnamon
1 teaspoon vanilla extract
**2 tablespoons FLEISCHMANN'S® Original
Margarine, divided**
**16 (4×1×1-inch) sticks day-old white
bread**
Powdered sugar, optional
Maple-flavored syrup, optional

In shallow bowl, combine Egg Beaters®, milk, cinnamon and vanilla.

In large nonstick griddle or skillet, over medium-high heat, melt 2 teaspoons margarine. Dip bread sticks in egg mixture to coat; transfer to griddle. Cook sticks on each side until golden, adding remaining margarine as needed.

Dust lightly with powdered sugar and serve with syrup, if desired.   *Makes 4 servings*

Nutrients per Serving: 4 French Toast Sticks

Calories 213	**Fiber** 1g
Fat 7g (sat 1g)	**Cholesterol** 1mg
Protein 10g	**Sodium** 431mg
Carbohydrate 25g	

Exchanges: 1-1/2 starch, 1 lean meat, 1 fat

Eggs Primavera

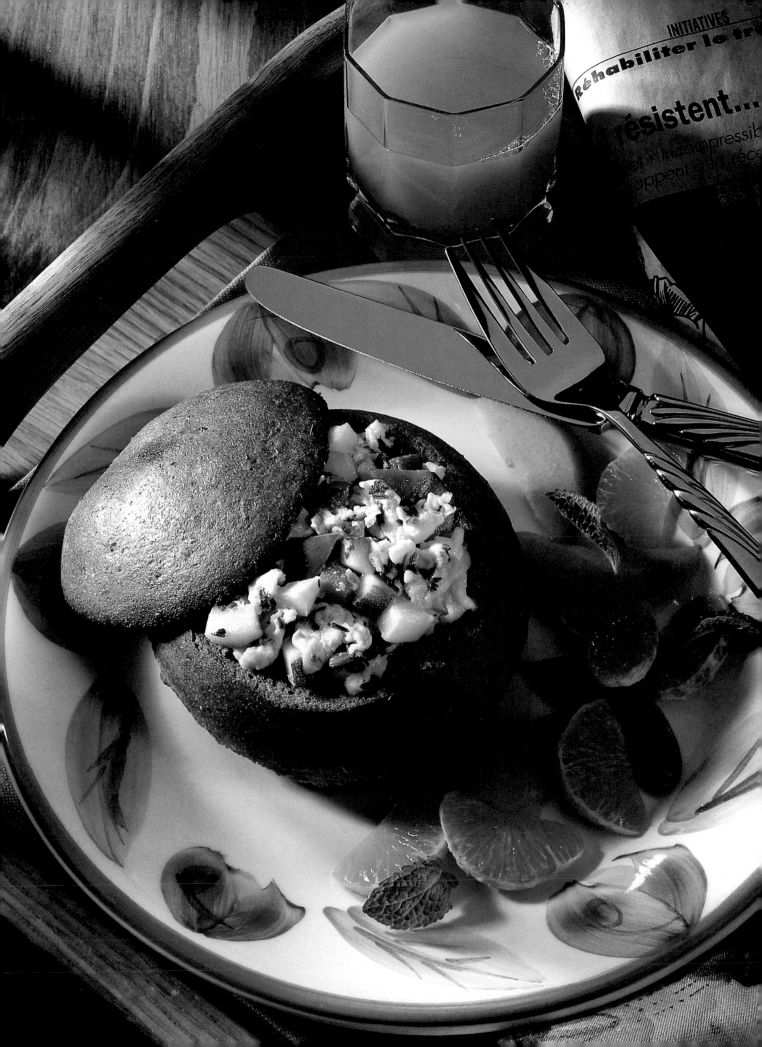

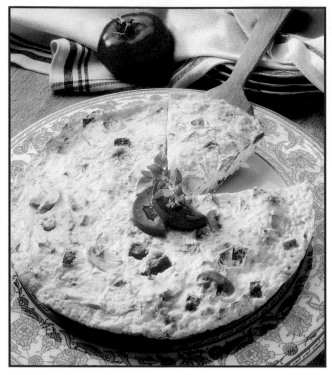

Zucchini Mushroom Frittata

Spray 10-inch ovenproof nonstick skillet lightly with nonstick cooking spray. Over medium-high heat, sauté zucchini, tomato and mushrooms in skillet until tender. Pour egg mixture into skillet, stirring well. Cover; cook over low heat for 15 minutes or until cooked on bottom and almost set on top. Remove lid and place skillet under broiler for 2 to 3 minutes or until desired doneness. Slide onto serving platter; cut into wedges to serve. Garnish with tomato slices and basil. *Makes 6 servings*

Nutrients per Serving: 1 Frittata wedge (1/6 of total recipe)

Calories 70	**Fiber** 1g
Fat 1g (sat 1g)	**Cholesterol** 5mg
Protein 9g	**Sodium** 316mg
Carbohydrate 5g	

Exchanges: 1 vegetable, 1 lean meat

Zucchini Mushroom Frittata

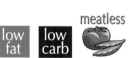

Quick Recipe　　　(Pictured above)

- **1-1/2 cups EGG BEATERS® Healthy Real Egg Product**
- **1/2 cup (2 ounces) shredded reduced-fat Swiss cheese**
- **1/4 cup fat-free (skim) milk**
- **1/2 teaspoon garlic powder**
- **1/4 teaspoon seasoned pepper**
  Nonstick cooking spray
- **1 medium zucchini, shredded (1 cup)**
- **1 medium tomato, chopped**
- **1 (4-ounce) can sliced mushrooms, drained**
  Tomato slices and fresh basil leaves, for garnish

In medium bowl, combine Egg Beaters®, cheese, milk, garlic powder and seasoned pepper; set aside.

O.J. Yogurt Shake

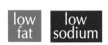

Quick Recipe

- **1 cup 2% low-fat milk**
- **1 carton (8 ounces) plain or vanilla low-fat yogurt**
- **1 can (6 ounces) frozen orange juice concentrate**
- **2 cups ice cubes, cracked**

Add milk, yogurt and orange juice concentrate to food processor or blender. Process until smooth and frothy. Add ice; process until smooth and frothy. *Makes 5 (1-cup) servings*

Favorite recipe from **Wisconsin Milk Marketing Board**

Nutrients per Serving: 1 Shake (1 cup)

Calories 107	**Fiber** <1g
Fat 2g (sat 1g)	**Cholesterol** 6mg
Protein 5g	**Sodium** 57mg
Carbohydrate 18g	

Exchanges: 1 fruit, 1/2 milk

Orange Cinnamon Pancakes

meatless

2 cups uncooked old-fashioned oats
2 cups orange juice
1/4 cup whole wheat pastry flour
1 teaspoon baking powder
1/2 teaspoon baking soda
1/2 teaspoon salt
1/2 teaspoon ground cinnamon
2 eggs, lightly beaten
1/4 cup canola oil
2 tablespoons honey
2 teaspoons grated orange peel
Plain fat-free yogurt and orange slices, for garnish (optional)

1. Combine oats and orange juice in large bowl. Cover and refrigerate overnight.

2. Just before cooking, sift flour, baking powder, baking soda, salt and cinnamon into oat mixture. Add eggs, oil, honey and orange peel; stir until just blended.

3. Coat large nonstick griddle or skillet with nonstick cooking spray. Heat over medium-low heat until hot.

4. For each pancake, spoon 1/4 cup batter onto hot griddle. Cook 2 to 3 minutes or until bubbles appear. Turn pancakes; cook until pancakes are lightly browned. Garnish with yogurt and orange slices, if desired.

Makes 12 pancakes, each 5 to 6 inches in diameter

Nutrients per Serving: 2 Pancakes

Calories 281	**Fiber** 3g
Fat 13g (sat 1g)	**Cholesterol** 71mg
Protein 7g	**Sodium** 403mg
Carbohydrate 37g	

Exchanges: 2-1/2 starch, 2 fat

Granola-Bran Muffins

1 cup boiling water
2-1/2 cups whole bran cereal
1 egg, lightly beaten
1 egg white
2 cups buttermilk
1/4 cup vegetable oil
1/2 cup finely chopped apple
2 cups all-purpose flour
1 cup sugar
1/2 cup quick-cooking rolled oats
1/2 cup wheat germ
2 teaspoons baking soda
1/2 teaspoon salt
1 cup raisins
1/2 cup chopped almonds, walnuts or pecans

Spray nonstick cooking spray in muffin cups or use paper liners. Preheat oven to 400°F. Pour boiling water over cereal in large bowl; cool. Stir in egg, egg white, buttermilk, oil and apple. Combine flour, sugar, oats, wheat germ, baking soda and salt in separate bowl. Stir in bran mixture. Stir in raisins and nuts. Fill prepared muffin cups 2/3 full. Bake 20 to 22 minutes or until wooden toothpick inserted into centers comes out clean. Remove from pans. Cool on wire racks. *Makes 36 muffins*

Favorite recipe from **Wisconsin Milk Marketing Board**

Nutrients per Serving: 1 Muffin

Calories 114	**Fiber** 2g
Fat 3g (sat <1g)	**Cholesterol** 6mg
Protein 3g	**Sodium** 160mg
Carbohydrate 20g	

Exchanges: 1 starch, 1 fat

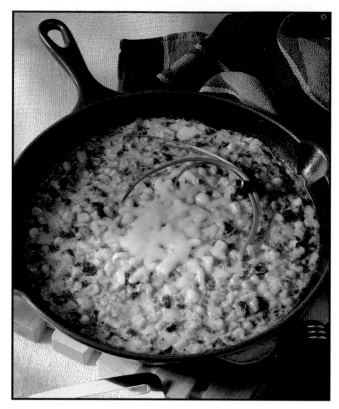

Spicy Mexican Frittata

Spicy Mexican Frittata

low fat | meatless

Quick Recipe   *(Pictured above)*

1 fresh jalapeño pepper*

1 clove garlic

1 medium tomato, peeled, halved, seeded and quartered

1/2 teaspoon ground coriander

1/2 teaspoon chili powder

   Nonstick cooking spray

1/2 cup chopped onion

1 cup frozen corn

6 egg whites

2 eggs

1/4 cup fat-free milk

1/4 teaspoon salt

1/4 teaspoon black pepper

1/4 cup (1 ounce) shredded part-skim farmer or mozzarella cheese

Jalapeño peppers can sting and irritate the skin; wear rubber gloves when handling peppers and do not touch eyes. Wash hands after handling peppers.

1. Add jalapeño pepper and garlic to food processor or blender. Process until finely chopped. Add tomato, coriander and chili powder. Cover; process until tomato is almost smooth.

2. Spray large nonstick skillet with cooking spray; heat skillet over medium heat until hot. Cook and stir onion until tender.

3. Add tomato mixture and corn to skillet; stir. Cook 3 to 4 minutes or until liquid is almost evaporated, stirring occasionally.

4. Combine egg whites, eggs, milk, salt and black pepper in medium bowl. Add egg mixture all at once to skillet. Cook, without stirring, 2 minutes or until eggs begin to set. Run large spoon around edge of skillet, lifting eggs for even cooking. Remove skillet from heat when eggs are almost set but surface is still moist.

5. Sprinkle with cheese. Cover; let stand 3 to 4 minutes or until surface is set and cheese is melted. Cut into 4 wedges.

Makes 4 servings

Nutrients per Serving: 1 Frittata wedge (1/4 of total recipe)

Calories 129	**Fiber** 2g
Fat 3g (sat 1g)	**Cholesterol** 108mg
Protein 12g	**Sodium** 371mg
Carbohydrate 14g	

Exchanges: 1/2 starch, 1 vegetable, 1 lean meat

Tip

To make a spicier dish, increase the jalapeño pepper and chili powder. This will not affect the nutritionals, only the heat level.

Mini Vegetable Quiches

meatless

(Pictured below)

- **2 cups cut-up vegetables (bell peppers, broccoli, zucchini and/or carrots)**
- **2 tablespoons chopped green onions**
- **2 tablespoons FLEISCHMANN'S® Original Margarine**
- **4 flour tortillas (8 inches), each cut into 8 triangles**
- **1 cup EGG BEATERS® Healthy Real Egg Product**
- **1 cup fat-free (skim) milk**
- **1/2 teaspoon dried basil leaves**

In medium nonstick skillet, over medium-high heat, sauté vegetables and green onions in margarine until tender.

Arrange 4 tortilla pieces in each of 8 (6-ounce) greased custard cups or ramekins, placing points of tortilla pieces at center of bottom of each cup and pressing lightly to form shape of cup. Divide vegetable mixture evenly among cups.

In small bowl, combine Egg Beaters®, milk and basil. Pour evenly over vegetable mixture.

Place cups on baking sheet. Bake at 375°F for 20 to 25 minutes or until puffed and knife inserted into centers comes out clean. Let stand 5 minutes before serving.   *Makes 8 servings*

Nutrients per Serving: 1 Mini Quiche

Calories 115	**Fiber** 1g
Fat 4g (sat 1g)	**Cholesterol** 1mg
Protein 6g	**Sodium** 184mg
Carbohydrate 14g	

Exchanges: 1/2 starch, 2 vegetable, 1/2 fat

Mini Vegetable Quiches

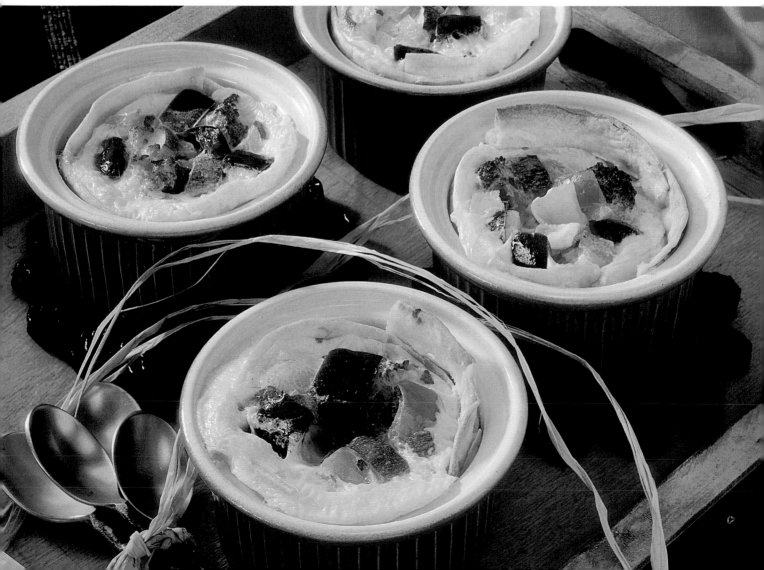

Western Omelet

Quick Recipe   *(Pictured at right)*

> **1/2 cup finely chopped red or green bell pepper**
>
> **1/3 cup cubed cooked potato**
>
> **2 slices turkey bacon, diced**
>
> **1/4 teaspoon dried oregano leaves**
>
> **2 teaspoons FLEISCHMANN'S® Original Margarine, divided**
>
> **1 cup EGG BEATERS® Healthy Real Egg Product**
>
> **Fresh oregano sprig, for garnish**

In 8-inch nonstick skillet, over medium heat, sauté bell pepper, potato, turkey bacon and dried oregano in 1 teaspoon margarine until tender. Remove from skillet; keep warm.

In same skillet, over medium heat, melt remaining margarine. Pour Egg Beaters® into skillet. Cook, lifting edges to allow uncooked portion to flow underneath.

When almost set, spoon vegetable mixture over half of omelet. Fold other half over vegetable mixture; slide onto serving plate. Garnish with fresh oregano.   *Makes 2 servings*

Nutrients per Serving: 1/2 of Omelet

Calories 166	**Fiber** 2g
Fat 6g (sat 1g)	**Cholesterol** 10mg
Protein 15g	**Sodium** 423mg
Carbohydrate 14g	

Exchanges: 1 starch, 2 lean meat

Apple Raisin Pancakes

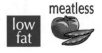

Quick Recipe

> **2 cups all-purpose flour**
>
> **2 tablespoons sugar**
>
> **1 tablespoon baking powder**
>
> **2 teaspoons ground cinnamon**
>
> **1-3/4 cups fat-free (skim) milk**
>
> **2/3 cup EGG BEATERS® Healthy Real Egg Product**
>
> **5 tablespoons FLEISCHMANN'S® Original Margarine, melted, divided**
>
> **3/4 cup chopped apple**
>
> **3/4 cup seedless raisins**

In large bowl, combine flour, sugar, baking powder and cinnamon. In medium bowl, combine milk, Egg Beaters® and 4 tablespoons margarine; stir into dry ingredients just until blended. Stir in apple and raisins.

Brush large nonstick griddle or skillet with some of remaining margarine; heat over medium-high heat.

Using 1/4 cup batter for each pancake, pour batter onto griddle. Cook until bubbly; turn and cook until lightly browned.

Repeat with remaining batter, using remaining margarine as needed, to make 16 pancakes.
     Makes 16 (4-inch) pancakes

Nutrients per Serving: 1 Pancake

Calories 133	**Fiber** 1g
Fat 3g (sat 1g)	**Cholesterol** <1mg
Protein 4g	**Sodium** 155mg
Carbohydrate 22g	

Exchanges: 1-1/2 starch, 1/2 fat

Western Omelet

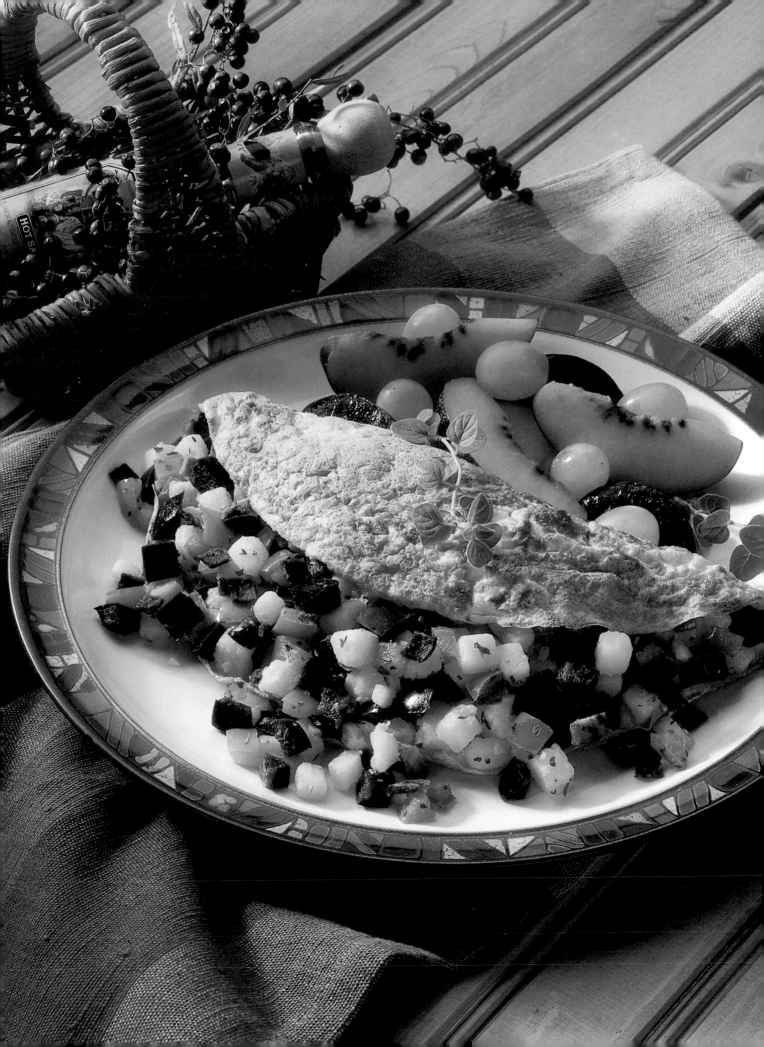

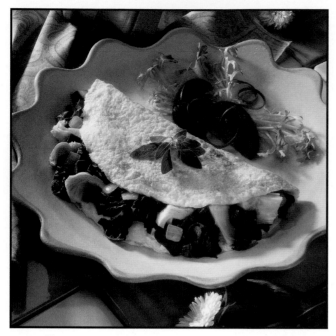

Greek Isles Omelet

over medium heat 5 to 7 minutes; as eggs begin to set, gently lift edges of omelet with spatula and tilt skillet so uncooked portion flows underneath.

4. When egg mixture is set, spoon vegetable mixture over half of omelet. Loosen omelet with spatula and fold in half. Slide omelet onto serving plate. Garnish, if desired.   *Makes 2 servings*

Nutrients per Serving: 1/2 of Omelet

Calories 111	**Fiber** 1g
Fat 3g (sat <1g)	**Cholesterol** 0mg
Protein 13g	**Sodium** 538mg
Carbohydrate 7g	

Exchanges: 1 vegetable, 2 lean meat

Greek Isles Omelet

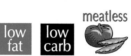

Quick Recipe   *(Pictured above)*

> **Nonstick cooking spray**
> **1/4 cup chopped onion**
> **1/4 cup canned artichoke hearts, rinsed and drained**
> **1/4 cup washed and torn spinach leaves**
> **1/4 cup chopped plum tomato**
> **1 cup cholesterol-free egg substitute**
> **2 tablespoons sliced pitted ripe olives, rinsed and drained**
> **Dash black pepper**

1. Spray small nonstick skillet with cooking spray; heat over medium heat until hot. Cook and stir onion 2 minutes or until crisp-tender.

2. Add artichoke hearts. Cook and stir until heated through. Add spinach and tomato; toss briefly. Remove from heat. Transfer vegetables to small bowl. Wipe out skillet and spray with cooking spray.

3. Combine egg substitute, olives and pepper in medium bowl. Heat skillet over medium heat until hot. Pour egg mixture into skillet. Cook

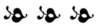

Potato & Onion Frittata

Quick Recipe

> **1 small baking potato, peeled, halved and sliced 1/8-inch thick (about 1/2 cup)**
> **1/4 cup chopped onion**
> **1 clove garlic, minced**
> **Dash ground black pepper**
> **1 tablespoon FLEISCHMANN'S® Original Margarine**
> **1 cup EGG BEATERS® Healthy Real Egg Product**

In 8-inch nonstick skillet, over medium-high heat, sauté potato, onion, garlic and pepper in margarine until tender. Pour Egg Beaters® evenly into skillet over potato mixture. Cook, without stirring, for 5 to 6 minutes or until cooked on bottom and almost set on top. Carefully turn frittata; cook for 1 to 2 minutes more or until done. Slide onto serving platter; cut into wedges to serve.   *Makes 2 servings*

Nutrients per Serving: 1 Frittata wedge (1/2 of total recipe)

Calories 179	**Fiber** 2g
Fat 5g (sat 1g)	**Cholesterol** 0mg
Protein 14g	**Sodium** 276mg
Carbohydrate 19g	

Exchanges: 1 starch, 1 lean meat, 1 fat

Scrambled Egg Burritos

meatless

Quick Recipe   (Pictured below)

Nonstick cooking spray
1 medium red bell pepper, chopped
5 green onions, sliced
1/2 teaspoon crushed red pepper flakes
1 cup cholesterol-free egg substitute *or* 8 egg whites
1 tablespoon chopped fresh cilantro or parsley
4 flour tortillas (8 inches)
1/2 cup (2 ounces) shredded reduced-fat Monterey Jack cheese
1/3 cup salsa

1. Spray medium nonstick skillet with cooking spray. Heat over medium heat until hot. Add bell pepper, green onions and red pepper flakes. Cook and stir 3 minutes or until vegetables are crisp-tender.

2. Add egg substitute to vegetables. Reduce heat to low. Cook and stir 3 minutes or until set. Sprinkle with cilantro.

3. Stack tortillas and wrap in paper towels. Microwave at HIGH 1 minute or until tortillas are hot.

4. Place one fourth of egg mixture on each tortilla. Sprinkle with 2 tablespoons cheese. Fold sides over to enclose filling. Serve with salsa.   *Makes 4 servings*

Nutrients per Serving: 1 Burrito with 1 tablespoon plus 1 teaspoon salsa

Calories 192	**Fiber** 2g
Fat 5g (sat 3g)	**Cholesterol** 10mg
Protein 13g	**Sodium** 423mg
Carbohydrate 23g	

Exchanges: 1 starch, 1 vegetable, 1-1/2 lean meat

Scrambled Egg Burrito

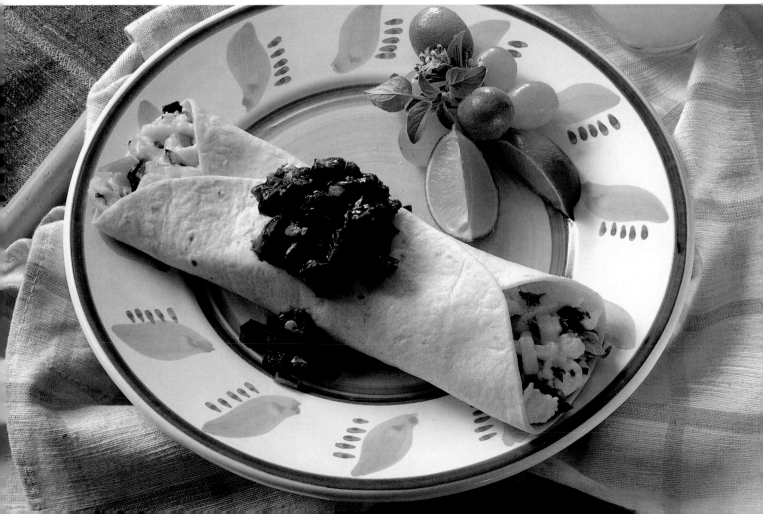

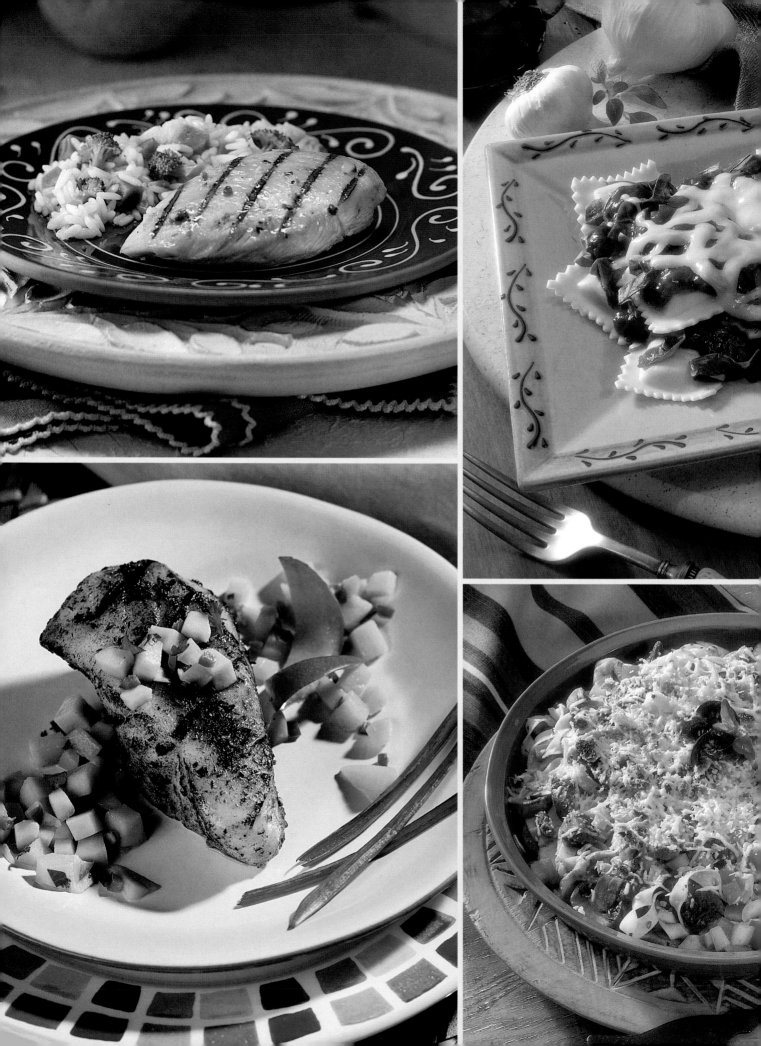

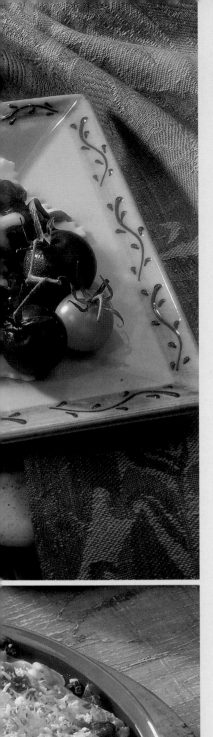

Main Dishes

❧ ❧ ❧

Grilled Chicken, Rice & Veggies

cooking for 1 or 2

(Pictured at left)

1 boneless skinless chicken breast (about 3 ounces)
3 tablespoons prepared reduced-fat Italian salad dressing, divided
1/2 cup fat-free reduced-sodium chicken broth
1/4 cup uncooked rice
1/2 cup frozen broccoli and carrot blend, thawed

1. Place chicken and 1 tablespoon salad dressing in resealable plastic food storage bag. Seal bag; turn to coat. Marinate in refrigerator 1 hour.

2. Remove chicken from marinade; discard marinade. Grill chicken over medium-hot coals 8 to 10 minutes or until chicken is no longer pink in center.

3. Meanwhile, bring broth to a boil in small saucepan; add rice. Cover; reduce heat and simmer 15 minutes, stirring in vegetables during last 5 minutes of cooking.

4. Remove from heat and stir in remaining 2 tablespoons dressing. Serve with chicken. *Makes 1 serving*

Nutrients per Serving: 1 Chicken breast with about 1-1/4 cups cooked Rice and Vegetable mixture

Calories 268	**Fiber** 4g
Fat 7g (sat 1g)	**Cholesterol** 54mg
Protein 26g	**Sodium** 516mg
Carbohydrate 25g	

Exchanges: 1-1/2 starch, 1 vegetable, 2-1/2 lean meat

Clockwise from top left: Grilled Chicken, Rice & Veggies, Ravioli with Homemade Tomato Sauce (page 78), Spicy Turkey Casserole (page 81) and Caribbean Sea Bass with Mango Salsa (page 85)

Spinach Lasagna

  meatless

(Pictured at right)

5 uncooked lasagna noodles
  Nonstick cooking spray

2 cups sliced fresh mushrooms

1 cup chopped onion

1 cup chopped green bell pepper

2 cloves garlic, minced

2 cans (8 ounces each) no-salt-added
  tomato sauce

1 teaspoon chopped fresh basil *or*
  1/4 teaspoon dried basil leaves

1 teaspoon chopped fresh oregano *or*
  1/4 teaspoon dried oregano leaves

1/4 teaspoon ground red pepper

1-1/2 cups low-fat (1%) cottage cheese or
  light ricotta cheese

1/4 cup grated Romano or Parmesan cheese

2 egg whites

3 tablespoons fine dry bread crumbs

1 package (10 ounces) frozen chopped
  spinach, thawed and well drained

3/4 cup (3 ounces) shredded part-skim
  mozzarella cheese

1/4 cup chopped fresh parsley

1. Prepare noodles according to package directions, omitting salt; drain. Rinse under cold water; drain. Set aside.

2. Coat large nonstick skillet with cooking spray. Add mushrooms, onion, bell pepper and garlic; cook and stir over medium heat until vegetables are tender. Stir in tomato sauce, basil, oregano and red pepper. Bring to a boil over medium-high heat. Reduce heat to medium-low. Simmer, uncovered, 10 minutes, stirring occasionally.

3. Preheat oven to 350°F. Combine cottage cheese, Romano cheese, egg whites and bread crumbs in medium bowl. Stir spinach into cottage cheese mixture. Cut noodles in half crosswise. Spread 1/2 cup tomato sauce in ungreased 8- or 9-inch square baking dish. Top with half the noodles, half the spinach mixture and half the remaining sauce. Repeat layers.

4. Cover and bake 45 minutes or until hot and bubbly. Sprinkle evenly with mozzarella cheese. Bake, uncovered, 2 to 3 minutes more or until cheese melts. Sprinkle evenly with parsley. Let stand 10 minutes. Cut into 4 wedges before serving. *Makes 4 servings*

Nutrients per Serving: 1 Lasagna wedge (1/4 of total recipe)

Calories 350	Fiber 7g
Fat 8g (sat 4g)	Cholesterol 23mg
Protein 30g	Sodium 746mg
Carbohydrate 40g	

Exchanges: 1 starch, 5 vegetable, 2-1/2 lean meat, 1/2 fat

Quick Pork Fajitas

Quick Recipe

1 pork tenderloin, about 1 pound, thinly
  sliced*

2 to 3 tablespoons fajita seasoning or
  marinade

1/2 onion, sliced

1/2 green bell pepper, sliced

4 to 6 flour tortillas (8 inches), warmed

*Placing pork tenderloin in freezer for about 20 minutes makes slicing easier.

In a shallow bowl, toss pork pieces with fajita seasoning. In large nonstick skillet over medium-high heat, stir-fry pork pieces with onion and green pepper until all is just tender. Wrap portions in flour tortillas with salsa. *Makes 4 servings*

*Favorite recipe from **National Pork Board***

Nutrients per Serving: 1 Fajita (without salsa)

Calories 276	Fiber 2g
Fat 8g (sat 3g)	Cholesterol 75mg
Protein 26g	Sodium 498mg
Carbohydrate 22g	

Exchanges: 1-1/2 starch, 3 lean meat

Spinach Lasagna

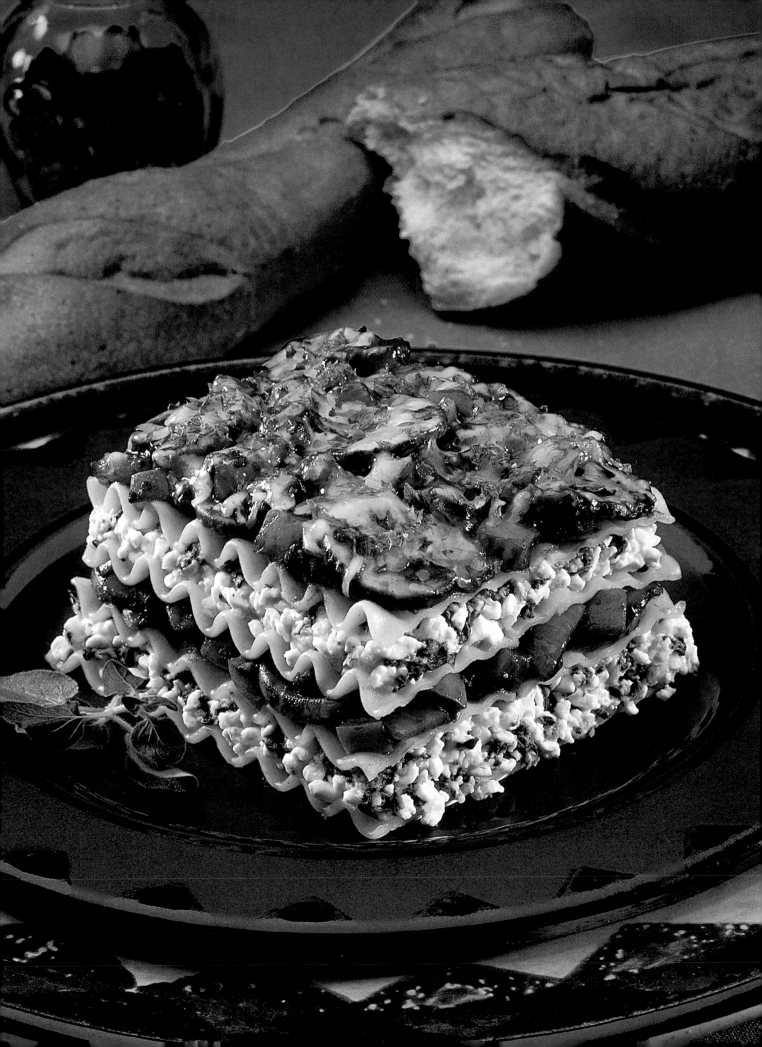

Ravioli with Homemade Tomato Sauce

meatless

(Pictured on page 74)

3 cloves garlic, peeled
1/2 cup fresh basil leaves
3 cups seeded quartered peeled tomatoes
2 tablespoons tomato paste
2 tablespoons prepared fat-free Italian salad dressing
1 tablespoon balsamic vinegar
1/4 teaspoon black pepper
1 package (9 ounces) refrigerated reduced-fat cheese ravioli
2 cups shredded washed spinach leaves
1 cup (4 ounces) shredded part-skim mozzarella cheese

Microwave Directions

1. To prepare tomato sauce, process garlic in food processor until coarsely chopped. Add basil; process until coarsely chopped. Add tomatoes, tomato paste, salad dressing, vinegar and pepper; process, using on/off pulsing action, until tomatoes are chopped.

2. Spray 9-inch square microwavable dish with nonstick cooking spray. Spread 1 cup tomato sauce in dish. Layer half of ravioli and spinach over tomato sauce. Repeat layers with 1 cup tomato sauce and remaining ravioli and spinach. Top with remaining 1 cup tomato sauce.

3. Cover with plastic wrap; refrigerate 1 to 8 hours. Vent plastic wrap. Microwave at MEDIUM (50% power) 20 minutes or until pasta is tender and hot. Sprinkle evenly with cheese. Microwave at HIGH 3 minutes or just until cheese melts. Let stand, covered, 5 minutes before serving.   *Makes 6 servings*

Note: This recipe was tested in an 1100-watt microwave oven.

Nutrients per Serving: 1/6 of total recipe

Calories 206	**Fiber** 3g
Fat 6g (sat 3g)	**Cholesterol** 40mg
Protein 13g	**Sodium** 401mg
Carbohydrate 26g	

Exchanges: 1 starch, 2 vegetable, 1 lean meat, 1/2 fat

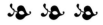

Chili Wagon Wheel Casserole

low fat   low sodium

8 ounces uncooked wagon wheel or other pasta
Nonstick cooking spray
1 pound 93% lean ground turkey or 95% lean ground beef
3/4 cup chopped green bell pepper
3/4 cup chopped onion
1 can (14-1/2 ounces) no-salt-added stewed tomatoes
1 can (8 ounces) no-salt-added tomato sauce
1/2 teaspoon black pepper
1/4 teaspoon ground allspice
1/2 cup (2 ounces) shredded reduced-fat Cheddar cheese

1. Preheat oven to 350°F. Cook pasta according to package directions, omitting salt. Drain and rinse; set aside.

2. Spray large nonstick skillet with cooking spray. Add ground turkey, bell pepper and onion; cook 5 minutes or until meat is no longer pink, stirring frequently. (Drain mixture if using ground beef.)

3. Stir in tomatoes, tomato sauce, black pepper and allspice; cook 2 minutes. Stir in pasta. Spoon mixture into 2-1/2-quart casserole. Sprinkle evenly with cheese. Bake, uncovered, 20 to 25 minutes or until heated through.
Makes 6 servings

Nutrients per Serving: 1-1/3 cups Casserole

Calories 290	**Fiber** 3g
Fat 3g (sat 1g)	**Cholesterol** 50mg
Protein 28g	**Sodium** 113mg
Carbohydrate 37g	

Exchanges: 2 starch, 1 vegetable, 2 lean meat

Jerked Pork Chops

Quick Recipe   *(Pictured below)*

- 2 teaspoons onion powder
- 1 teaspoon sugar
- 1 teaspoon dried thyme leaves, crushed
- 1/2 teaspoon salt
- 1/2 teaspoon ground allspice
- 1/2 teaspoon ground red pepper
- 1/4 teaspoon ground nutmeg
- Nonstick cooking spray
- 4 boneless pork loin chops, cut 1/2 inch thick (about 1 pound), trimmed of fat
- 4 cups cooked white rice
- 2 green onions, chopped

1. Combine onion powder, sugar, thyme, salt, allspice, ground red pepper and nutmeg in small bowl; mix well. Rub both sides of pork chops with spice mixture.

2. Spray nonstick skillet with cooking spray; heat over medium heat. Cook pork chops about 5 minutes per side or until juicy and barely pink in center.

3. Serve pork chops over rice; sprinkle with green onions. Garnish with red onion and scented geranium leaf, if desired.

Makes 4 servings

Nutrients per Serving: 1 Pork Chop with 1 cup cooked rice

Calories 375	**Fiber** 1g
Fat 6g (sat 2g)	**Cholesterol** 62mg
Protein 29g	**Sodium** 335mg
Carbohydrate 47g	

Exchanges: 3 starch, 3 lean meat

Jerked Pork Chop

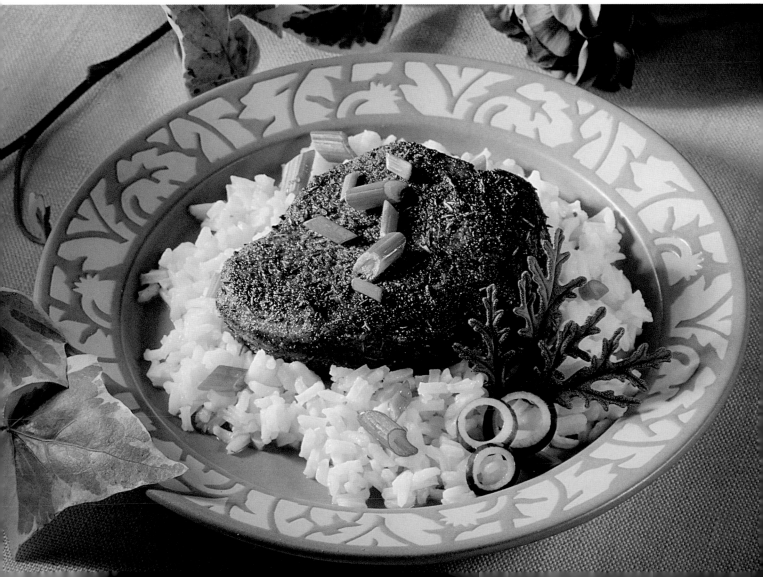

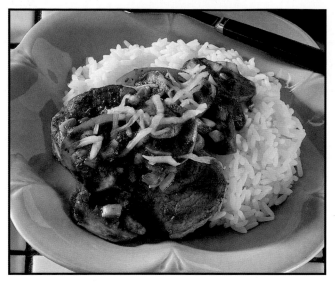

Italian Pork Cutlets

Italian Pork Cutlets

(Pictured above)

1 teaspoon CRISCO® Oil*
6 (4 ounces each) lean, boneless center-cut pork loin slices, 3/4 inch thick
1 can (8 ounces) tomato sauce
1-1/2 cups sliced fresh mushrooms
1 small green bell pepper, cut into strips
1/2 cup sliced green onions with tops
1 teaspoon Italian seasoning
1/2 teaspoon salt
1/8 teaspoon black pepper
1/4 cup water
1 teaspoon cornstarch
1/2 cup (2 ounces) shredded low moisture part-skim mozzarella cheese
3 cups hot cooked rice (cooked without salt or fat)

Use your favorite Crisco Oil product.

1. Heat oil in large skillet on medium heat. Add meat. Cook until browned on both sides.

2. Add tomato sauce, mushrooms, green bell pepper, onions, Italian seasoning, salt and black pepper. Reduce heat to low. Cover. Simmer 30 minutes or until meat is tender.

3. Combine water and cornstarch in small bowl. Stir until well blended. Add to juices in skillet. Cook and stir until thickened.

4. Sprinkle cheese over meat mixture. Cover. Heat until cheese melts. Serve with rice.

Makes 6 servings

Nutrients per Serving: 1 Pork Cutlet with 1/2 cup sauce and 1/2 cup rice

Calories 314	**Fiber** 1g
Fat 8g (sat 3g)	**Cholesterol** 77mg
Protein 30g	**Sodium** 544mg
Carbohydrate 28g	

Exchanges: 1 starch, 2-1/2 vegetable, 3 lean meat

Quick Skillet Quiche

meatless

Quick Recipe

4 eggs
1/3 cup 1% milk
2 teaspoons Cajun seasoning
1 cup reduced-fat Cheddar cheese, divided
1 cup UNCLE BEN'S® Instant Rice
1 cup chopped fresh asparagus
3/4 cup chopped green onions
1/2 cup chopped red bell pepper

1. Preheat oven to 350°F. In medium bowl, whisk eggs, milk, Cajun seasoning and 1/2 cup cheese.

2. Cook rice according to package directions. Meanwhile, spray medium skillet with nonstick cooking spray. Heat over medium heat until hot. Add asparagus, green onions and bell pepper. Cook and stir 5 minutes. Add rice and mix well.

3. Shape rice mixture to form crust on bottom and halfway up side of skillet. Pour egg mixture over crust. Sprinkle with remaining 1/2 cup cheese. Cover; cook over medium-low heat 10 minutes or until eggs are nearly set. Transfer skillet to oven and bake 5 minutes or until eggs are completely set. *Makes 6 servings*

Nutrients per Serving: 1 Quiche wedge (1/6 of total recipe)

Calories 173	**Fiber** 1g
Fat 6g (sat 3g)	**Cholesterol** 152mg
Protein 11g	**Sodium** 372mg
Carbohydrate 17g	

Exchanges: 1 starch, 1 vegetable, 1 lean meat, 1/2 fat

Spicy Turkey Casserole

(Pictured on page 74)

- 1 tablespoon olive oil
- 1 pound turkey breast cutlets, cut into 1/2-inch pieces
- 2 spicy chicken or turkey sausages (3 ounces each), sliced 1/2 inch thick
- 1 cup diced green bell pepper
- 1/2 cup sliced mushrooms
- 1/2 cup diced onion
- 1 jalapeño pepper,* seeded and minced (optional)
- 1/2 cup fat-free reduced-sodium chicken broth or water
- 1 can (14 ounces) no-salt-added diced tomatoes, undrained
- 1 teaspoon Italian seasoning
- 1/4 teaspoon black pepper
- 1/2 teaspoon paprika
- 1 cup cooked yolk-free egg noodles
- 6 tablespoons grated Parmesan cheese
- 2 tablespoons coarse bread crumbs

Jalapeño peppers can sting and irritate the skin; wear rubber gloves when handling peppers and do not touch eyes. Wash hands after handling peppers.

1. Preheat oven to 350°F.

2. Heat oil in large nonstick skillet. Add turkey and sausages; cook and stir over medium heat 2 minutes. Add bell pepper, mushrooms, onion and jalapeño pepper, if desired. Cook and stir 5 minutes. Add chicken broth; cook 1 minute, scraping any browned bits off bottom of skillet. Add tomatoes with juice, seasonings and noodles.

3. Spoon turkey mixture into shallow 10-inch round casserole. Sprinkle evenly with cheese and bread crumbs. Bake 15 to 20 minutes or until mixture is hot and bread crumbs are brown.   *Makes 6 servings*

Nutrients per Serving: 1 cup Casserole

Calories 268	**Fiber** 3g
Fat 6g (sat 2g)	**Cholesterol** 52mg
Protein 25g	**Sodium** 347mg
Carbohydrate 23g	

Exchanges: 1 starch, 1 vegetable, 3 lean meat

Peppercorn Beef Kabobs

low carb

Quick Recipe   (Pictured below)

- 1 pound boneless beef sirloin steak, cut 1 inch thick
- 1-1/2 teaspoons black peppercorns, crushed
- 1 clove garlic, minced
- 1/2 teaspoon salt
- 1/2 teaspoon paprika
- 1 medium onion, cut into 12 wedges
- Cherry tomato halves (optional)

1. Cut beef into 1-inch pieces. Combine peppercorns, garlic, salt and paprika in shallow dish. Add beef; toss to coat.

2. Thread an equal number of beef pieces onto each of 4 (12-inch) skewers, along with 3 onion wedges. (If using bamboo skewers, soak in water 25 to 30 minutes before using, to prevent them from burning.) Place kabobs on rack in broiler pan. Broil 3 to 4 inches from heat 9 to 12 minutes, turning occasionally. Garnish with tomatoes, if desired.   *Makes 4 servings*

Nutrients per Serving: 1 Kabob

Calories 158	**Fiber** 1g
Fat 4g (sat 2g)	**Cholesterol** 54mg
Protein 25g	**Sodium** 339mg
Carbohydrate 3g	

Exchanges: 3 lean meat

Peppercorn Beef Kabobs

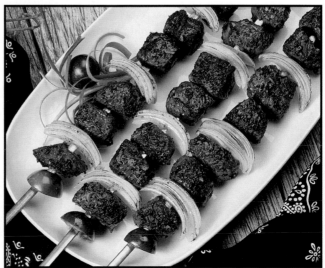

Sesame Chicken and Vegetable Stir-Fry

Quick Recipe   *(Pictured at right)*

- 1 tablespoon dark sesame oil
- 1 pound chicken tenders, cut into 1-inch pieces
- 2 cups broccoli florets
- 1 small red bell pepper, sliced
- 1/2 cup onion slices (about 1 small)
- 1/2 cup snow peas
- 1 can (8 ounces) sliced water chestnuts, drained
- 2 cloves garlic, minced
- 1 teaspoon Chinese five-spice powder
- 1 cup fat-free reduced-sodium chicken broth
- 2 teaspoons cornstarch
- 2 tablespoons cold water
- 2 cups hot cooked white rice

1. Heat sesame oil in wok or large nonstick skillet over medium heat until hot. Add chicken; stir-fry about 8 minutes or until chicken is no longer pink in center. Remove from wok.

2. Add broccoli, bell pepper, onion, snow peas, water chestnuts and garlic to wok; stir-fry 5 to 8 minutes or until vegetables are crisp-tender. Sprinkle with five-spice powder; cook and stir 1 minute.

3. Return chicken to wok. Add chicken broth; heat to a boil. Combine cornstarch and water in small bowl; stir into broth mixture. Boil 1 to 2 minutes, stirring constantly. Serve over rice.

Makes 4 servings

Nutrients per Serving: 2 cups Chicken mixture with 1/2 cup cooked rice

Calories 304	**Fiber** 4g
Fat 5g (sat 1g)	**Cholesterol** 48mg
Protein 28g	**Sodium** 396mg
Carbohydrate 38g	

Exchanges: 2 starch, 1 vegetable, 2-1/2 lean meat

New England Fisherman's Skillet

Quick Recipe

- 4 small red potatoes, diced
- 1 medium onion, chopped
- 1 tablespoon olive oil
  Herb seasoning mix to taste (optional)
- 2 stalks celery, chopped
- 2 cloves garlic, minced
- 1/2 teaspoon dried thyme, crushed
- 1 can (14-1/2 ounces) DEL MONTE® Stewed Tomatoes - Original Recipe
- 1 pound firm white fish (such as halibut, snapper or cod), cut into bite-size chunks

1. Brown potatoes and onion in oil over medium-high heat in large skillet, stirring occasionally. Season with herb seasoning mix, if desired.

2. Stir in celery, garlic and thyme; cook 4 minutes. Add tomatoes; bring to a boil. Cook 4 minutes or until thickened.

3. Add fish; cover and cook over medium heat 5 to 8 minutes or until fish flakes easily with fork.

4. Garnish with lemon wedges and chopped parsley, if desired.   *Makes 4 servings*

Nutrients per Serving: 1-1/4 cups New England Fisherman's Skillet

Calories 241	**Fiber** 3g
Fat 6g (sat 1g)	**Cholesterol** 36mg
Protein 26g	**Sodium** 403mg
Carbohydrate 22g	

Exchanges: 1 starch, 1 vegetable, 3 lean meat

Sesame Chicken and Vegetable Stir-Fry

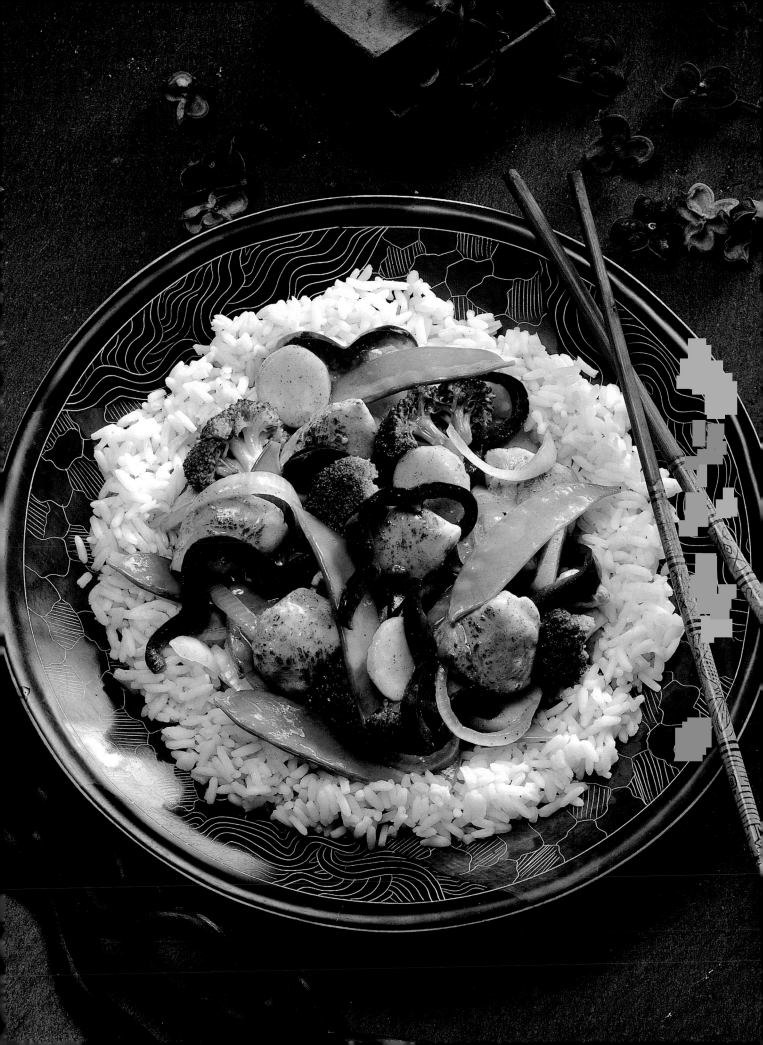

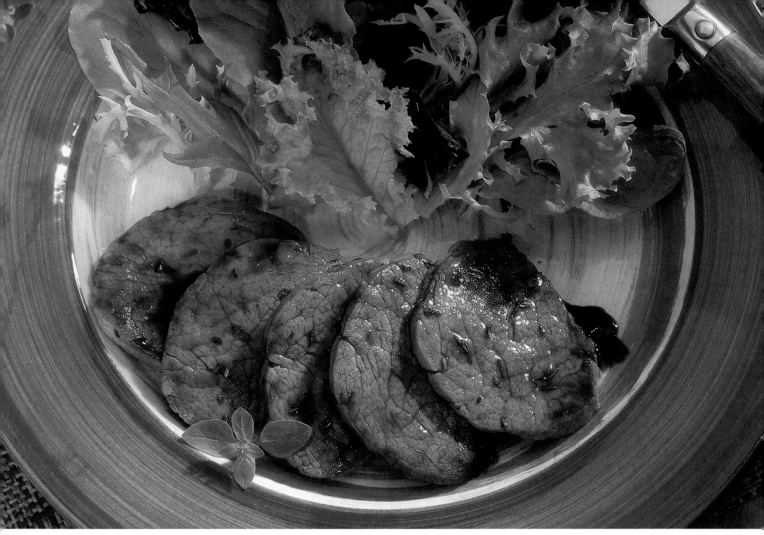

Blackberry-Glazed Pork Medallions

Blackberry-Glazed Pork Medallions

low carb

Quick Recipe

1/3 cup no-sugar-added seedless blackberry spread

4-1/2 teaspoons red wine vinegar or cider vinegar

1 tablespoon sugar

1/4 teaspoon red pepper flakes

    Nonstick cooking spray

1 teaspoon canola oil

1 pound pork tenderloin, cut into 1/4-inch-thick slices

1/4 teaspoon dried thyme leaves, divided

1/4 teaspoon salt, divided

1. Whisk blackberry spread, vinegar, sugar and red pepper flakes in small bowl until blended; set aside.

2. Coat large nonstick skillet with cooking spray. Heat over medium-high heat until hot. Add oil and tilt skillet to coat bottom. Add half of pork slices; sprinkle with half of thyme and half of salt. Cook 2 minutes; turn and cook 1 minute on other side. Remove pork from skillet; set aside. Repeat with remaining pork, thyme and salt. Remove pork; set aside.

3. Add blackberry mixture to skillet; bring to a boil over high heat. Add reserved pork slices, discarding any accumulated juices. Cook about 4 minutes, turning constantly, until pork is richly glazed. Garnish, if desired.

Makes 4 servings

Nutrients per Serving: 1/4 of total recipe

Calories 186	**Fiber** <1g
Fat 5g (sat 2g)	**Cholesterol** 66mg
Protein 23g	**Sodium** 219mg
Carbohydrate 10g	

Exchanges: 1/2 fruit, 3 lean meat

Caribbean Sea Bass with Mango Salsa

Quick Recipe   *(Pictured on page 74)*

4 skinless sea bass fillets (4 ounces each), about 1 inch thick

1 teaspoon Caribbean jerk seasoning
  Nonstick cooking spray

1 ripe mango *or* **2 medium peaches, peeled, pitted and diced,** *or* **1 cup diced drained bottled mango**

2 tablespoons chopped fresh cilantro

2 teaspoons fresh lime juice

1 teaspoon minced fresh or bottled jalapeño pepper*

*Jalapeño peppers can sting and irritate the skin; wear rubber gloves when handling peppers and do not touch eyes. Wash hands after handling peppers.

1. Prepare grill or preheat broiler.

2. Sprinkle fish with seasoning; coat lightly with cooking spray. Grill fish over medium coals or broil 5 inches from heat 4 to 5 minutes per side or until fish flakes easily when tested with fork.

3. Meanwhile, combine mango, cilantro, lime juice and jalapeño pepper in small bowl; mix well. Serve over fish.   *Makes 4 servings*

Nutrients per Serving: 1 fillet with about 1/4 cup Mango Salsa

Calories 146	**Fiber** 1g
Fat 3g (sat 1g)	**Cholesterol** 47mg
Protein 21g	**Sodium** 189mg
Carbohydrate 9g	

Exchanges: 1/2 fruit, 2 lean meat

Tip

Beef, full of high-quality protein and also an important source of dietary iron and zinc, can easily fit into a healthy meal plan. Try to choose lean cuts, ones with "loin" or "round" in the name. Sirloin, tenderloin and top round are some of the leanest cuts.

Beef and Broccoli

Quick Recipe

1 pound lean beef tenderloin

2 teaspoons minced fresh ginger *or* **1/2 teaspoon ground ginger**

2 cloves garlic, minced

1/2 teaspoon canola oil

3 cups broccoli florets

1/4 cup water

2 tablespoons bottled teriyaki sauce

2 cups hot cooked white rice
  Red bell pepper strips, for garnish (optional)

1. Cut beef across the grain into 1/8-inch-thick slices; cut each slice into 1-1/2-inch pieces. Toss beef with ginger and garlic in medium bowl.

2. Heat oil in wok or large nonstick skillet over medium heat. Add beef mixture; stir-fry 3 to 4 minutes or until beef is barely pink in center. Remove and reserve.

3. Add broccoli and water to wok; cover and steam 3 to 5 minutes or until broccoli is crisp-tender.

4. Return beef and any accumulated juices to wok. Add teriyaki sauce. Cook until heated through.

5. Serve over rice. Garnish with red bell pepper strips, if desired.   *Makes 4 servings*

Nutrients per Serving: 1/4 of Beef and Broccoli mixture with 1/2 cup cooked rice

Calories 392	**Fiber** 3g
Fat 11g (sat 4g)	**Cholesterol** 95mg
Protein 37g	**Sodium** 393mg
Carbohydrate 34g	

Exchanges: 2 starch, 1 vegetable, 4 lean meat

Meatballs in Creamy Mustard Sauce

cooking for 1 or 2

6 ounces 95% lean ground beef

1/3 cup fresh bread crumbs

2 tablespoons chopped green onion with tops

1 tablespoon plus 1 teaspoon Dijon mustard, divided

1/2 teaspoon lemon pepper

1/4 teaspoon salt

3 ounces uncooked fettuccine *or* 1-1/4 cups uncooked tricolor rotini pasta

1/2 cup fat-free reduced-sodium beef broth

2 teaspoons cornstarch

3 tablespoons reduced-fat sour cream

Minced fresh parsley (optional)

1. Preheat oven to 400°F. Spray broiler pan with nonstick cooking spray.

2. Combine beef, bread crumbs, green onion, 1 tablespoon mustard, lemon pepper and salt in small bowl. Shape into 8 meatballs. Place in single layer on prepared broiler pan. Bake, uncovered, 15 minutes or until no longer pink in center.

3. Meanwhile, cook fettuccine according to package directions, omitting salt. Drain and keep warm.

4. Whisk together beef broth, remaining 1 teaspoon mustard and cornstarch in medium saucepan until smooth. Cook over low heat, stirring constantly, until mixture comes to a boil. Remove from heat. Stir about 1 tablespoon broth mixture into sour cream. Stir sour cream mixture into broth mixture in saucepan. Heat over low heat 1 minute. *Do not boil.* Remove from heat; stir in meatballs. Serve immediately.

5. Divide fettuccine evenly between 2 serving plates and top with meatballs and sauce. Garnish with parsley, if desired.

Makes 2 servings

Nutrients per Serving: 3/4 cup cooked fettuccine with 1/2 of Meatballs and Sauce

Calories 318	**Fiber** 2g
Fat 8g (sat 3g)	**Cholesterol** 52mg
Protein 24g	**Sodium** 657mg
Carbohydrate 37g	

Exchanges: 2-1/2 starch, 2-1/2 lean meat

Spring Lamb Skillet

Quick Recipe

2 teaspoons olive oil

1 pound boneless lamb, cut into 1-inch cubes

2 cups thinly sliced yellow squash

2 cups (about 8 ounces) sliced fresh mushrooms

2 medium tomatoes, seeded and chopped

1/2 cup sliced green onions

3 cups cooked brown rice

1/2 teaspoon dried rosemary

1/2 teaspoon salt

1/2 teaspoon cracked black pepper

Heat oil in large skillet over medium heat until hot. Add lamb and cook 3 to 5 minutes or until lamb is browned. Remove from skillet; reserve. Add squash, mushrooms, tomatoes and onions to skillet; cook 2 to 3 minutes or until vegetables are tender. Stir in rice, rosemary, salt, pepper and reserved lamb. Cook until heated through.

Makes 6 servings

Favorite recipe from **USA Rice Federation**

Nutrients per Serving: about 1 cup Spring Lamb Skillet

Calories 261	**Fiber** 3g
Fat 8g (sat 2g)	**Cholesterol** 52mg
Protein 20g	**Sodium** 254mg
Carbohydrate 27g	

Exchanges: 1 starch, 2 vegetable, 2 lean meat, 1/2 fat

Marinated Chicken and Pesto Pizza

Quick Recipe   *(Pictured below)*

- **8 ounces chicken tenders**
- **1/4 cup prepared fat-free Italian salad dressing**
- **Nonstick cooking spray**
- **1/2 cup sun-dried tomatoes**
- **1 cup chopped plum tomatoes**
- **1 tablespoon prepared pesto**
- **1 teaspoon salt-free Italian herb blend**
- **1/4 teaspoon red pepper flakes**
- **1 (12-inch) prepared pizza crust**
- **1 cup (4 ounces) shredded part-skim mozzarella cheese**

1. Cut chicken tenders into 2×1/2-inch strips. Place in large resealable plastic food storage bag. Pour Italian dressing over chicken. Seal bag and turn to coat. Marinate at room temperature 15 minutes, turning several times.

2. Remove chicken from marinade; discard marinade. Spray large nonstick skillet with cooking spray; heat over medium heat until hot. Add chicken; cook and stir 5 minutes or until no longer pink in center.

3. Meanwhile, cover sun-dried tomatoes with boiling water in small bowl; let stand 10 minutes. Drain; cut tomatoes into 1/4-inch strips.

4. Preheat oven to 450°F. Combine plum tomatoes, pesto, herb blend and red pepper flakes in small bowl. Spread onto pizza crust. Add chicken tenders and sun-dried tomatoes; sprinkle cheese evenly over top.

5. Bake 8 to 10 minutes or until cheese melts and pizza is heated through. Cut pizza into 6 wedges before serving.   *Makes 6 servings*

Nutrients per Serving: 1 Pizza wedge (1/6 of total recipe)

Calories 322	**Fiber** 3g
Fat 10g (sat 1g)	**Cholesterol** 30mg
Protein 16g	**Sodium** 512mg
Carbohydrate 38g	

Exchanges: 2 starch, 1 vegetable, 2 lean meat, 1/2 fat

Marinated Chicken and Pesto Pizza

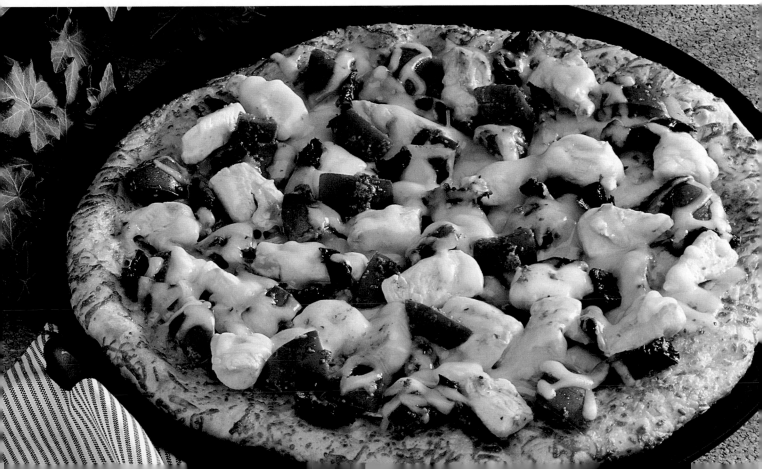

Chicken Primavera

Quick Recipe (Pictured at right)

2 tablespoons CRISCO® Oil*

6 boneless, skinless chicken breast halves, cut into 1-inch pieces (about 1-1/2 pounds chicken)

1 clove garlic, minced

3 cups broccoli flowerets

2 cups sliced fresh mushrooms

1 fresh tomato, chopped

1 package (8 ounces) spaghetti or linguine, cooked and well drained

3/4 cup grated Parmesan cheese

1 tablespoon dried basil leaves

1/2 teaspoon salt

1/4 teaspoon pepper

3/4 cup evaporated skimmed milk

Use your favorite Crisco Oil product.

1. Heat oil in large skillet on medium-high heat. Add chicken and garlic. Cook and stir 5 minutes or until chicken is no longer pink in center. Remove to serving plate.

2. Add broccoli, mushrooms and tomato to skillet. Cook and stir 3 to 5 minutes or until broccoli is crisp-tender. Return chicken to skillet to heat.

3. Transfer mixture to large serving bowl. Add spaghetti, Parmesan cheese, basil, salt and pepper. Toss to mix. Add milk. Mix lightly. Serve immediately on spinach-covered plates, if desired. *Makes 6 servings*

Nutrients per Serving: 1-1/3 cups Chicken Primavera (without spinach)

Calories 401	**Fiber** 3g
Fat 10g (sat 3g)	**Cholesterol** 75mg
Protein 40g	**Sodium** 507mg
Carbohydrate 37g	

Exchanges: 2 starch, 1 vegetable, 4 lean meat

Paella

Nonstick cooking spray

10 ounces boneless skinless chicken breasts

1 teaspoon canola oil

1/2 cup uncooked white rice

4 cloves garlic, finely chopped

1/2 cup sliced onion

1/2 cup sliced green bell pepper

1 cup fat-free reduced-sodium chicken broth

1/2 teaspoon ground turmeric

1/4 teaspoon salt

1/4 teaspoon paprika

1/4 teaspoon black pepper

1/2 cup frozen green peas

1/2 cup drained canned diced tomatoes

8 ounces raw medium shrimp, peeled and deveined

1. Preheat oven to 350°F.

2. Spray large nonstick skillet with cooking spray; heat over medium-high heat until hot. Add chicken. Cook 10 minutes or until chicken is no longer pink in center, turning once. Remove chicken from skillet. Cool 10 minutes or until cool enough to handle. Cut into 1-inch pieces.

3. Heat oil in large ovenproof skillet or paella pan over medium heat until hot. Add rice and garlic. Cook 5 minutes or until rice is browned, stirring occasionally. Add onion and bell pepper. Stir in chicken broth, turmeric, salt, paprika and black pepper. Stir in peas and tomatoes. Place chicken and shrimp on top of rice mixture.

4. Bake, covered, 20 minutes or until heated through. Let stand 5 minutes before serving. *Makes 4 servings*

Nutrients per Serving: 1-1/4 cups Paella

Calories 276	**Fiber** 2g
Fat 3g (sat 1g)	**Cholesterol** 127mg
Protein 32g	**Sodium** 522mg
Carbohydrate 27g	

Exchanges: 1 starch, 2 vegetable, 3 lean meat

Chicken Primavera

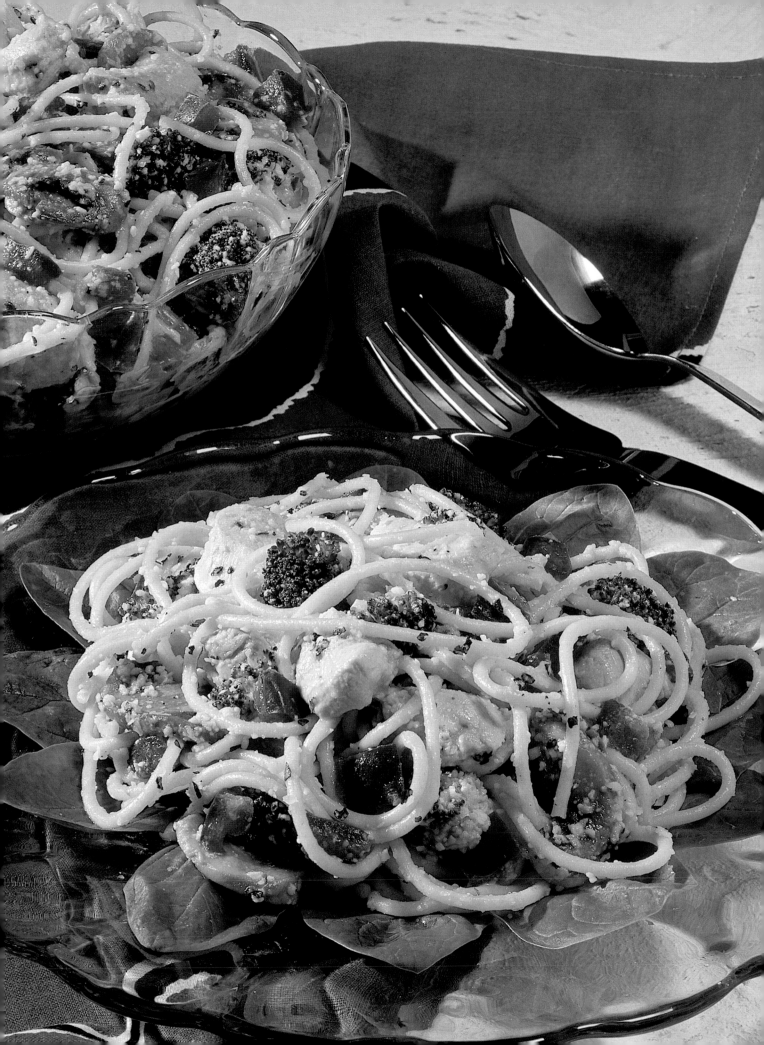

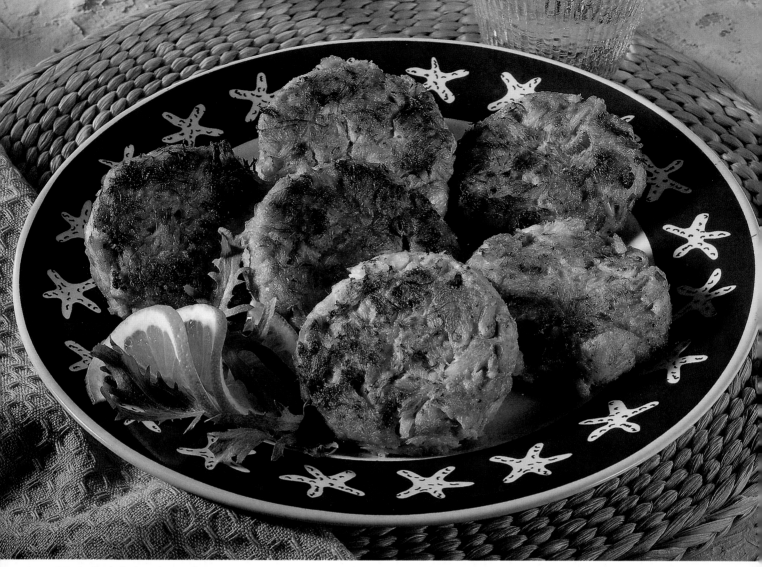

Maryland Crab Cakes

Maryland Crab Cakes

low carb

(Pictured above)

1 pound fresh backfin crabmeat, cartilage removed

10 reduced-sodium crackers (2 inches each), crushed to equal 1/2 cup crumbs

1 rib celery, finely chopped

1 green onion, finely chopped

1/4 cup cholesterol-free egg substitute

3 tablespoons fat-free tartar sauce

1 teaspoon seafood seasoning

2 teaspoons canola oil

1. Combine crabmeat, cracker crumbs, celery and onion in medium bowl; set aside.

2. Mix egg substitute, tartar sauce and seafood seasoning in small bowl; pour over crabmeat mixture. Gently mix so large lumps will not be broken. Shape into 6 (3/4-inch-thick) patties. Cover; refrigerate 30 minutes.

3. Spray large nonstick skillet with nonstick cooking spray. Add oil; heat over medium-high heat. Place crab cakes in skillet; cook 3 to 4 minutes on each side or until cakes are lightly browned. Garnish with lemon wedges or slices, if desired. *Makes 6 servings*

Nutrients per Serving: 1 Crab Cake

Calories 127	**Fiber** 0g
Fat 4g (sat 0g)	**Cholesterol** 44mg
Protein 14g	**Sodium** 382mg
Carbohydrate 8g	

Exchanges: 1/2 starch, 1-1/2 lean meat

Beef and Pineapple Kabobs

1 pound boneless beef top sirloin steak or beef top round steak, cut 1 inch thick
1 small onion, finely chopped
1/2 cup bottled reduced-sodium teriyaki sauce
16 pieces (1-inch cubes) fresh pineapple
1 can (8 ounces) water chestnuts, drained

1. Cut steak into 1/4-inch-thick strips. For marinade, combine onion and teriyaki sauce in small bowl. Add beef strips, stirring to coat.

2. Alternately thread beef strips (weaving back and forth), pineapple cubes and water chestnuts onto 4 bamboo or thin metal skewers. (If using bamboo skewers, soak in water 25 to 30 minutes before using, to prevent them from burning.)

3. Place kabobs on grid over medium coals. Grill 4 minutes, turning once, or until meat is cooked through. Serve immediately.

Makes 4 servings

Serving Suggestion: Serve with hot cooked rice and stir-fried broccoli, mushrooms and red bell peppers.

Nutrients per Serving: 1 Kabob (without rice and stir-fried vegetables)

Calories 232	**Fiber** 1g
Fat 7g (sat 3g)	**Cholesterol** 101mg
Protein 38g	**Sodium** 880mg
Carbohydrate 26g	

Exchanges: 1 fruit, 1 vegetable, 4 lean meat

Tip

If you can't find a 9-ounce package frozen cut green beans at your grocery store, use half of a 16-ounce package for the Vegetable Pork Skillet.

Vegetable Pork Skillet

high fiber

1 tablespoon CRISCO® Oil*
4 (4 ounces *each*) lean, boneless, center-cut pork loin chops, 1/2 inch thick
2 medium onions, thinly sliced and separated into rings
1 can (14-1/2 ounces) whole tomatoes, undrained
3/4 cup water
2 teaspoons paprika
1 teaspoon salt
1/2 teaspoon celery seed
1/4 teaspoon pepper
1/4 teaspoon garlic powder
1 pound unpeeled potatoes (about 3 medium), chopped
1 package (9 ounces) frozen cut green beans

*Use your favorite Crisco Oil product.

1. Heat oil in large skillet on medium heat. Add meat. Cook until browned on both sides. Remove from skillet.

2. Add onions to skillet. Cook and stir until tender. Add tomatoes, water, paprika, salt, celery seed, pepper and garlic powder. Bring to a boil.

3. Return meat to skillet. Reduce heat to low. Cover. Simmer 15 minutes.

4. Add potatoes. Cover. Simmer 15 minutes.

5. Add beans. Cover. Simmer 5 to 7 minutes or until potatoes and beans are tender.

Makes 4 servings

Nutrients per Serving: 1 Pork chop with 1-1/2 cups Vegetables

Calories 351	**Fiber** 6g
Fat 11g (sat 3g)	**Cholesterol** 62mg
Protein 29g	**Sodium** 800mg
Carbohydrate 34g	

Exchanges: 2 starch, 1 vegetable, 3 lean meat

Chili Beef & Red Pepper Fajitas with Chipotle Salsa

high fiber

cooking for 1 or 2

Quick Recipe *(Pictured at right)*

6 ounces top sirloin steak, thinly sliced
1/2 medium lime
1-1/2 teaspoons chili powder
1/2 teaspoon ground cumin
1/2 cup diced plum tomatoes
1/4 cup mild picante sauce
1/2 canned chipotle chili pepper in adobo sauce *or* 1 teaspoon chopped canned jalapeño pepper
Nonstick cooking spray
1/2 cup sliced onion
1/2 medium red bell pepper, cut into thin strips
2 fat-free flour tortillas (10 inches), warmed
1/4 cup fat-free sour cream
2 tablespoons chopped fresh cilantro leaves (optional)

1. Place steak on plate. Squeeze lime over top; sprinkle with chili powder and cumin. Toss to coat well; let stand 10 minutes.

2. Meanwhile, to prepare salsa, combine tomatoes and picante sauce in small bowl. Place chipotle on small plate. Using fork, mash completely. Stir mashed chipotle into tomato mixture. Set salsa aside.

3. Coat 12-inch nonstick skillet with cooking spray. Heat over high heat until hot. Add onion and bell pepper; cook and stir 3 minutes or until tender; remove from skillet. Lightly spray skillet with cooking spray. Add beef; cook and stir 1 minute. Return onion and bell pepper to skillet; cook 1 minute longer.

4. Place 1/2 the beef mixture in center of each tortilla; fold up sides over filling. Top each fajita with 1/4 cup prepared salsa, 2 tablespoons sour cream and cilantro, if desired.

Makes 2 servings

Note: For a less spicy salsa, use less chipotle chili or eliminate it completely.

92 *Main Dishes*

Nutrients per Serving: 1 Fajita with 1/4 cup Salsa and 2 tablespoons sour cream

Calories 245	**Fiber** 9g
Fat 4g (sat 2g)	**Cholesterol** 45mg
Protein 21g	**Sodium** 530mg
Carbohydrate 31g	

Exchanges: 1 starch, 2 vegetable, 2 lean meat

❧ ❧ ❧

Chicken Cacciatore Over Pasta

low fat

Quick Recipe

16 ounces skinned and boned uncooked chicken breast, cut into 32 pieces
1/2 cup chopped onion
1/2 cup chopped green bell pepper
2 cups (one 16-ounce can) tomatoes, chopped and drained
1 cup (one 8-ounce can) tomato sauce
2 tablespoons SPLENDA® Granular
1-1/2 teaspoons Italian seasoning
1/3 cup sliced ripe olives
1/8 teaspoon black pepper
3 cups hot cooked noodles or any favorite pasta, rinsed and drained

In large skillet sprayed with olive oil-flavored nonstick cooking spray, sauté chicken, onion and green pepper for 6 to 8 minutes. Stir in undrained tomatoes and tomato sauce. Add SPLENDA® Granular, Italian seasoning, olives, and black pepper. Mix well to combine. Lower heat and simmer for 10 to 15 minutes, stirring occasionally. For each serving, place 1/2 cup pasta on plate and spoon 2/3 cup sauce over top.

Makes 6 servings

Nutrients per Serving: 1/2 cup pasta with 2/3 cup sauce

Calories 239	**Fiber** 3g
Fat 3g (sat 1g)	**Cholesterol** 70mg
Protein 23g	**Sodium** 297mg
Carbohydrate 29g	

Exchanges: 2 starch, 2 lean meat

Chili Beef & Red Pepper Fajita with Chipotle Salsa

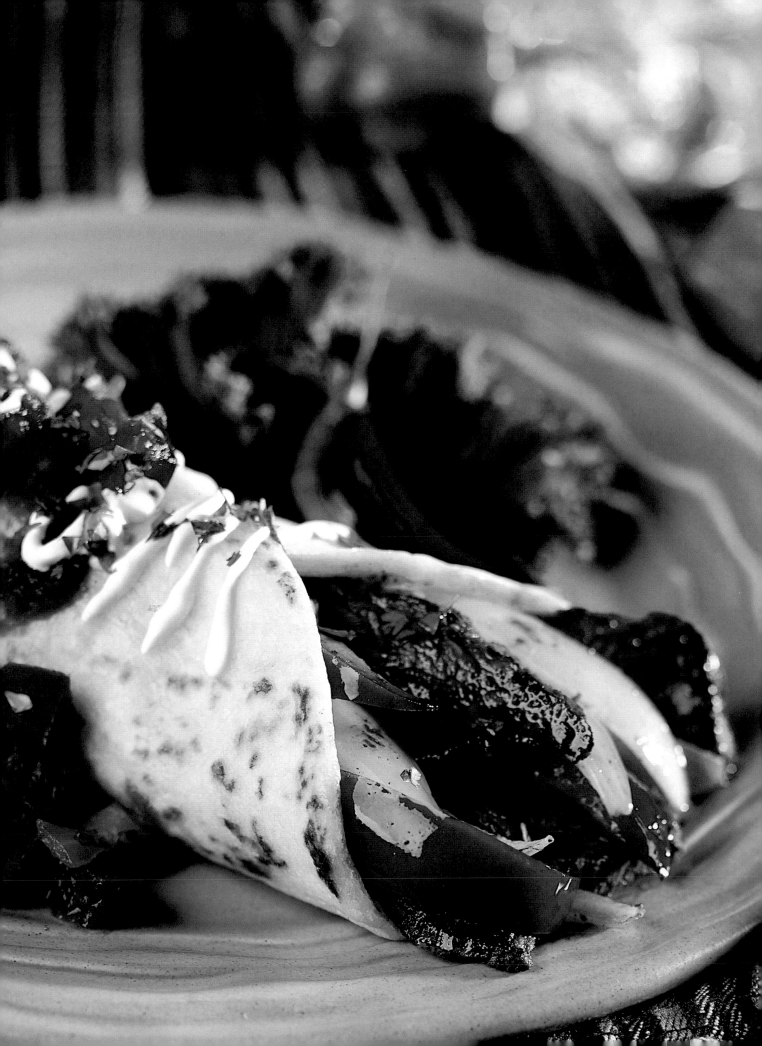

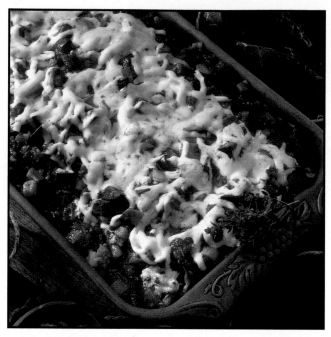

Cannelloni with Tomato-Eggplant Sauce

Cannelloni with Tomato-Eggplant Sauce

meatless

(Pictured above)

1 package (10 ounces) fresh spinach
1 cup fat-free ricotta cheese
4 egg whites, beaten
1/4 cup (1 ounce) grated Parmesan cheese
2 tablespoons finely chopped fresh parsley
1/2 teaspoon salt (optional)
8 manicotti (about 4 ounces uncooked), cooked and cooled
  Tomato-Eggplant Sauce (recipe follows)
1 cup (4 ounces) shredded reduced-fat mozzarella cheese

1. Preheat oven to 350°F.

2. Wash spinach; do not pat dry. Place spinach in saucepan; cook, covered, over medium-high heat 3 to 5 minutes or until spinach is wilted. Cool slightly and drain; chop finely.

3. Combine ricotta cheese, spinach, egg whites, Parmesan cheese, parsley and salt, if desired, in large bowl; mix well. Spoon mixture into cooked manicotti shells; arrange in 13×9-inch

baking dish. Spoon Tomato-Eggplant Sauce over manicotti; sprinkle evenly with mozzarella cheese.

4. Bake manicotti, uncovered, 25 to 30 minutes or until hot and bubbly.
Makes 4 servings (2 manicotti each)

Tomato-Eggplant Sauce

Olive oil-flavored nonstick cooking spray
1 small eggplant, coarsely chopped
1/2 cup chopped onion
2 cloves garlic, minced
1/2 teaspoon dried tarragon leaves
1/4 teaspoon dried thyme leaves
1 can (16 ounces) no-salt-added whole tomatoes, undrained, coarsely chopped
  Salt (optional)
  Black pepper (optional)

1. Spray large nonstick skillet with cooking spray; heat over medium heat until hot. Add eggplant, onion, garlic, tarragon and thyme; cook and stir about 5 minutes or until vegetables are tender.

2. Stir in tomatoes with juice; bring to a boil. Reduce heat and simmer, uncovered, 3 to 4 minutes. Season to taste with salt and pepper, if desired. *Makes about 2-1/2 cups*

Nutrients per Serving: 2 filled manicotti shells with about 1/2 cup Sauce and 1/4 cup mozzarella cheese

Calories 338	**Fiber** 3g
Fat 7g (sat 4g)	**Cholesterol** 26mg
Protein 30g	**Sodium** 632mg
Carbohydrate 40g	

Exchanges: 1-1/2 starch, 3 vegetable, 3 lean meat

Tip

Prevent the manicotti from becoming too soft by slightly undercooking the pasta shells before cooling and then stuffing them with the spinach-cheese mixture.

Tuscan Chicken Breasts with Polenta

(Pictured below right)

4 cups fat-free reduced-sodium chicken broth
1 cup yellow cornmeal
   Nonstick cooking spray
1/2 teaspoon garlic powder
1/2 teaspoon dried Italian seasoning
1/4 teaspoon salt
1/4 teaspoon black pepper
8 skinless chicken breasts (about 3 pounds)
   Fresh spinach leaves, steamed (optional)
   Tuscan Tomato Sauce (recipe follows)

1. Heat chicken broth to a boil in large nonstick saucepan; slowly stir in cornmeal. Reduce heat to low; cook, stirring frequently, 15 to 20 minutes or until mixture is very thick and pulls away from side of pan. Spray 9×5-inch loaf pan with cooking spray. (Mixture may be lumpy.) Pour polenta into prepared pan. Cool; refrigerate 2 to 3 hours or until firm.

2. Preheat oven to 350°F. Combine garlic powder, Italian seasoning, salt and pepper in small bowl; rub on all surfaces of chicken.

3. Arrange chicken, breast sides up, in single layer in 13×9-inch baking pan. Bake, uncovered, about 45 minutes or until chicken is no longer pink in center and juices run clear.

4. Remove polenta from pan; transfer to cutting board. Cut polenta crosswise into 16 slices. Cut slices into triangles, if desired.

5. Spray large nonstick skillet with cooking spray; heat over medium heat until hot. Cook polenta about 4 minutes per side or until lightly browned.

6. Place spinach leaves, if desired, on serving plates. Arrange polenta slices and chicken over spinach; top with Tuscan Tomato Sauce.

Makes 8 servings

Tuscan Tomato Sauce

   Nonstick cooking spray
1/2 cup chopped onion
2 cloves garlic, minced
8 plum tomatoes, coarsely chopped
1 can (8 ounces) tomato sauce
2 teaspoons dried basil leaves
2 teaspoons dried oregano leaves
2 teaspoons dried rosemary leaves, crushed
1/2 teaspoon black pepper

Spray medium nonstick saucepan with cooking spray; heat over medium heat until hot. Add onion and garlic; cook and stir about 5 minutes or until tender. Stir in remaining ingredients; heat to a boil. Reduce heat to low and simmer, uncovered, about 6 minutes or until desired consistency is reached, stirring occasionally.

Makes about 3 cups

Nutrients per Serving: 1 Chicken Breast with 2 slices Polenta (4 triangles) and 1/4 cup plus 2 tablespoons Tuscan Tomato Sauce

Calories 248	**Fiber** 4g
Fat 4g (sat 1g)	**Cholesterol** 69mg
Protein 31g	**Sodium** 406mg
Carbohydrate 21g	

Exchanges: 1 starch, 1 vegetable, 3 lean meat

Tuscan Chicken Breast with Polenta

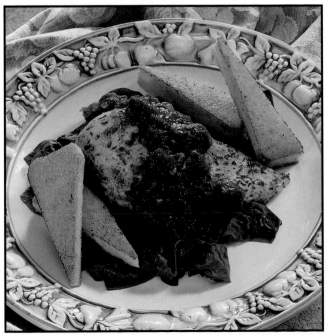

Mushroom Pasta Scampi

`high fiber`

Quick Recipe   *(Pictured at right)*

> **8 ounces uncooked linguine**
> **2 tablespoons olive oil**
> **1 pound fresh white mushrooms, sliced**
> **1 tablespoon chopped garlic**
> **1 pound frozen peeled and deveined raw large shrimp, thawed***
> **10 ounces fresh spinach, trimmed and torn into pieces (about 7 cups)**
> **1/4 cup grated Parmesan cheese**
> **1/4 teaspoon crushed red pepper**

*To quickly thaw shrimp: Place in a colander with cold running water for about 8 minutes; drain thoroughly.

Cook linguine according to package directions. Drain, reserving 1/2 cup pasta water; set aside. Meanwhile, heat olive oil in large nonstick skillet. Add mushrooms and garlic; cook and stir about 5 minutes or until tender and mushroom liquid is almost evaporated. Add shrimp; cover and cook about 5 minutes or until shrimp is almost cooked through. Stir in spinach and reserved 1/2 cup pasta water, if desired. Cover and cook about 1 minute or until spinach is wilted. Place pasta in serving bowl; stir in mushroom and shrimp mixture, Parmesan cheese and red pepper. Toss to combine. Season with salt, if desired.   *Makes 4 servings*

Favorite recipe from **Mushroom Council**

Nutrients per Serving: 1-1/2 cups Scampi (without salt seasoning)

Calories 415	**Fiber** 9g
Fat 13g (sat 3g)	**Cholesterol** 240mg
Protein 37g	**Sodium** 370mg
Carbohydrate 38g	

Exchanges: 2 starch, 1 vegetable, 4 lean meat, 1/2 fat

Chicken with Rosemary-Peach Glaze

Quick Recipe

> **4 boneless skinless chicken breasts (about 1 pound)**
> **2 tablespoons reduced-sodium soy sauce, divided**
> **1/3 cup peach preserves**
> **1 sprig fresh rosemary *or* 1 teaspoon dried rosemary leaves, crushed**
> **1 tablespoon lemon juice**
> **1 clove garlic, minced**
> **2 cups cooked wild rice and long-grain rice mix**

1. Preheat broiler. Spray baking sheet with nonstick cooking spray.

2. Sprinkle chicken evenly with 1 tablespoon soy sauce; place on prepared baking sheet. Broil 4 to 6 inches from heat 3 minutes; turn and broil 3 minutes.

3. Meanwhile, combine preserves, rosemary, lemon juice, remaining 1 tablespoon soy sauce and garlic in small saucepan. Cook over medium-low heat 5 minutes.

4. Brush sauce over chicken; broil 2 minutes. Turn and brush with sauce. Broil 2 minutes longer or until chicken is no longer pink in center. Discard any remaining sauce. Serve chicken with rice.   *Makes 4 servings*

Nutrients per Serving: 1 breast with 1/2 cup cooked rice mix

Calories 280	**Fiber** <1g
Fat 6g (sat 1g)	**Cholesterol** 69mg
Protein 29g	**Sodium** 761mg
Carbohydrate 25g	

Exchanges: 1 starch, 1/2 fruit, 3 lean meat

Mushroom Pasta Scampi

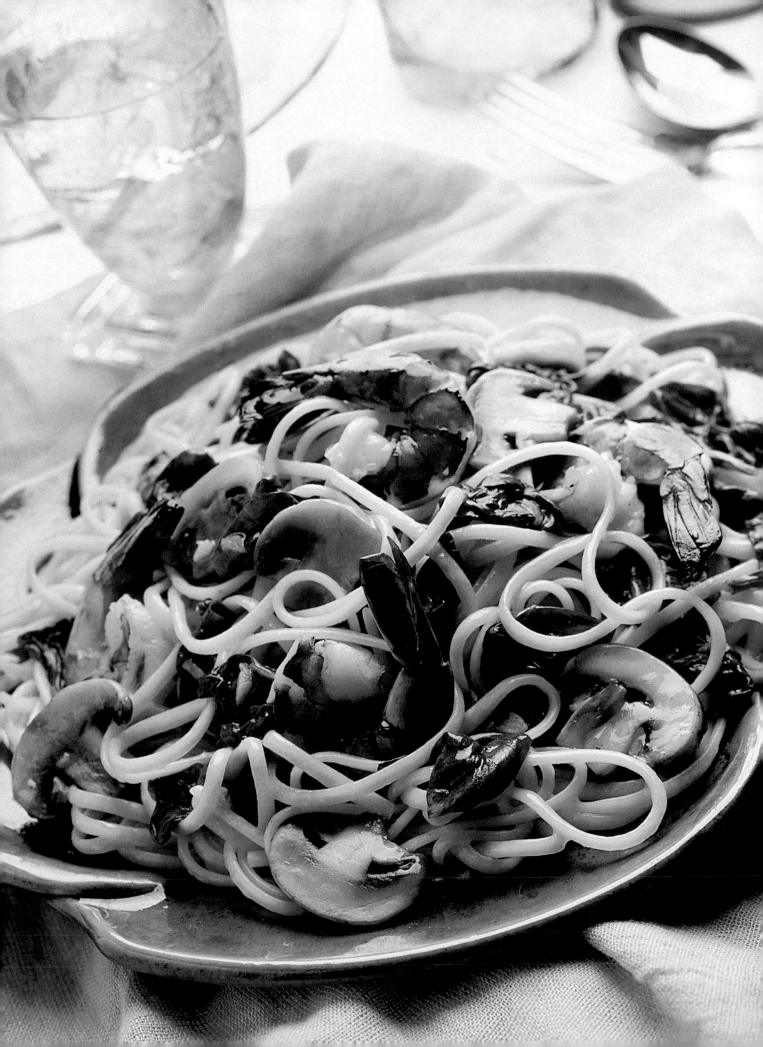

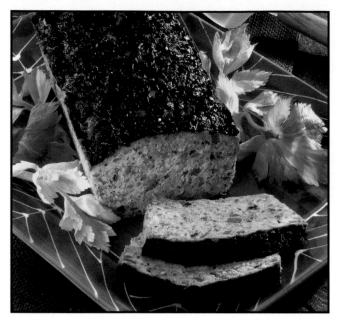

Turkey Meat Loaf

Turkey Meat Loaf

(Pictured above)

> **1 tablespoon canola oil**
> **3/4 cup chopped onion**
> **1/2 cup chopped celery**
> **1 clove garlic, minced**
> **2/3 cup fat-free reduced-sodium chicken broth or water**
> **1/2 cup uncooked bulgur**
> **1/2 cup cholesterol-free egg substitute**
> **1 tablespoon reduced-sodium soy sauce**
> **1/4 teaspoon ground cumin**
> **1/4 teaspoon paprika**
> **1/4 teaspoon black pepper**
> **8 tablespoons chili sauce, divided**
> **1 pound 93% lean ground turkey**

1. Heat oil in medium skillet. Add onion, celery and garlic. Cook and stir 3 minutes over low heat. Add broth and bulgur. Bring to a boil. Reduce heat to low. Cover and simmer 10 to 15 minutes or until bulgur is tender and all liquid is absorbed. Transfer to large bowl; cool to lukewarm.

2. Preheat oven to 375°F. Stir egg substitute, soy sauce, cumin, paprika and pepper into bulgur. Add 6 tablespoons chili sauce and ground turkey. Stir well until blended.

3. Pat turkey mixture into 8×4-inch loaf pan coated with nonstick cooking spray. Top with remaining 2 tablespoons chili sauce.

4. Bake meat loaf about 45 minutes or until browned and juices run clear. Let stand 10 minutes. Remove from pan; cut into 10 slices.   *Makes 5 servings (2 slices each)*

Nutrients per Serving: 2 slices Meat Loaf

Calories 197	**Fiber** 4g
Fat 5g (sat <1g)	**Cholesterol** 36mg
Protein 20g	**Sodium** 437mg
Carbohydrate 18g	

Exchanges: 1 starch, 1 vegetable, 2 lean meat

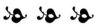

Salmon with Dill-Mustard Sauce

Quick Recipe

> **2 tablespoons fresh lemon juice**
> **2 tablespoons fresh lime juice**
> **4 salmon fillets (4 ounces each)**
> **1/4 cup fat-free mayonnaise**
> **1 tablespoon Dijon mustard**
> **1 tablespoon chopped fresh dill**
> **Dill sprigs (optional)**

1. Combine lemon juice and lime juice in glass baking dish. Rinse salmon; pat dry. Place salmon in juices; marinate 10 minutes, turning once.

2. Meanwhile, combine mayonnaise, mustard and 1 tablespoon dill in small bowl; set aside.

3. Preheat broiler. Spray rack of broiler pan with nonstick cooking spray. Remove salmon from juices; pat dry. Discard juices. Place salmon on rack. Broil 4 inches from heat 3 to 4 minutes on each side or until salmon flakes in center. Serve salmon with prepared sauce. Garnish with dill sprigs, if desired.   *Makes 4 servings*

Nutrients per Serving: 1 Salmon fillet with about 1 tablespoon Sauce

Calories 220	**Fiber** <1g
Fat 12g (sat 3g)	**Cholesterol** 74mg
Protein 23g	**Sodium** 260mg
Carbohydrate 3g	

Exchanges: 3 lean meat, 1 fat

Red Snapper Vera Cruz

low fat | low sodium | low carb

Quick Recipe   *(Pictured below)*

4 red snapper fillets (4 ounces each)
1/4 cup fresh lime juice
1 tablespoon fresh lemon juice
1 teaspoon chili powder
4 green onions with 4 inches of tops,
   sliced in 1/2-inch lengths
1 medium tomato, coarsely chopped
1/2 cup chopped Anaheim or green bell
   pepper
1/2 cup chopped red bell pepper
   Black pepper

1. Place red snapper in shallow 9- to 10-inch round microwavable baking dish. Combine lime juice, lemon juice and chili powder in small bowl. Pour over snapper. Marinate 10 minutes, turning once or twice.

2. Sprinkle green onions, tomato, Anaheim and bell pepper over snapper. Season to taste with black pepper. Cover dish loosely with vented plastic wrap. Microwave at HIGH 5 to 6 minutes or just until snapper flakes in center, rotating dish every 2 minutes. Let stand, covered, 4 minutes.   *Makes 4 servings*

Note: This recipe was tested in an 1100-watt microwave oven.

Nutrients per Serving: 1 fillet with about 1/2 cup salsa

Calories 144
Fat 2g (sat <1g)
Protein 24g
Carbohydrate 7g
Fiber 2g
Cholesterol 42mg
Sodium 61mg

Exchanges: 1 vegetable, 2-1/2 lean meat

Red Snapper Vera Cruz

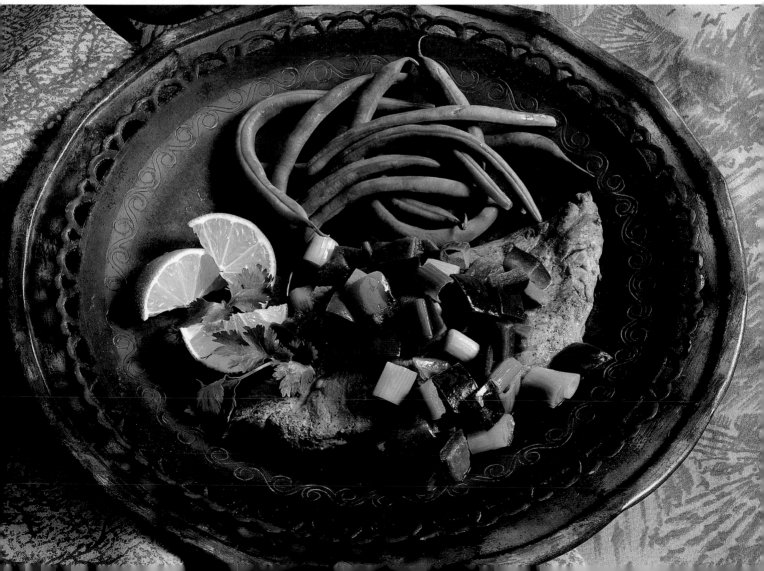

Fusilli Pizzaiola with Turkey Meatballs

low sodium

1 pound 93% lean ground turkey
1 egg, lightly beaten
1 tablespoon fat-free milk
1/4 cup Italian-seasoned dry bread crumbs
2 tablespoons chopped fresh parsley
1/4 teaspoon black pepper, divided
1/2 cup chopped onion
1/2 cup grated carrots
1 clove garlic, minced
2 teaspoons olive oil
2 cans (14-1/2 ounces each) no-salt-added diced tomatoes, undrained
2 tablespoons chopped fresh basil *or* 2 teaspoons dried basil leaves
1 tablespoon no-salt-added tomato paste
1/2 teaspoon dried thyme leaves
1 bay leaf
8 ounces uncooked fusilli or other spiral-shaped pasta

1. Preheat oven to 350°F. Combine turkey, egg and milk in medium bowl. Add bread crumbs, parsley and 1/8 teaspoon black pepper; mix well. With wet hands, shape turkey mixture into 24 (1-inch) meatballs.

2. Spray baking sheet with nonstick cooking spray. Arrange meatballs on baking sheet. Bake 25 minutes or until no longer pink in center.

3. Place onion, carrots, garlic and oil in medium saucepan. Cook and stir over high heat 5 minutes or until onion is tender. Add tomatoes, basil, tomato paste, thyme, bay leaf and remaining 1/8 teaspoon black pepper. Bring to a boil; reduce heat to low. Simmer 25 minutes; add meatballs. Cover; simmer 5 to 10 minutes or until sauce thickens slightly. Remove bay leaf.

4. Meanwhile, cook pasta according to package directions, omitting salt. Drain well. Place in large serving bowl. Spoon meatballs and sauce evenly over pasta. Garnish, if desired.

Makes 4 servings

Nutrients per Serving: 1 cup cooked pasta with 1-1/4 cups Meatballs and sauce (6 Meatballs)

Calories 333	**Fiber** 3g
Fat 10g (sat 2g)	**Cholesterol** 116mg
Protein 21g	**Sodium** 111mg
Carbohydrate 39g	

Exchanges: 2 starch, 2 vegetable, 2 lean meat, 1/2 fat

Skillet Chicken Pot Pie

Quick Recipe   *(Pictured at right)*

1 can (10-3/4 ounces) fat-free reduced-sodium cream of chicken soup, undiluted
1-1/4 cups fat-free milk, divided
1 package (10 ounces) frozen mixed vegetables
2 cups diced cooked chicken
1/2 teaspoon black pepper
1 cup buttermilk biscuit baking mix
1/4 teaspoon summer savory or parsley (optional)

1. Heat soup, 1 cup milk, vegetables, chicken and pepper in medium skillet over medium heat until mixture comes to a boil.

2. Combine biscuit mix and summer savory, if desired, in small bowl. Stir in 3 to 4 tablespoons milk just until soft batter is formed. Drop batter by tablespoonfuls onto chicken mixture to make 6 dumplings. Partially cover; simmer 12 minutes or until dumplings are cooked through, spooning liquid from pot pie over dumplings once or twice during cooking. Garnish with additional summer savory, if desired.   *Makes 6 servings*

Nutrients per Serving: 1/2 cup Chicken mixture with 1 dumpling

Calories 241	**Fiber** <1g
Fat 5g (sat 1g)	**Cholesterol** 33mg
Protein 17g	**Sodium** 422mg
Carbohydrate 25g	

Exchanges: 1 starch, 1-1/2 vegetable, 2 lean meat

Skillet Chicken Pot Pie

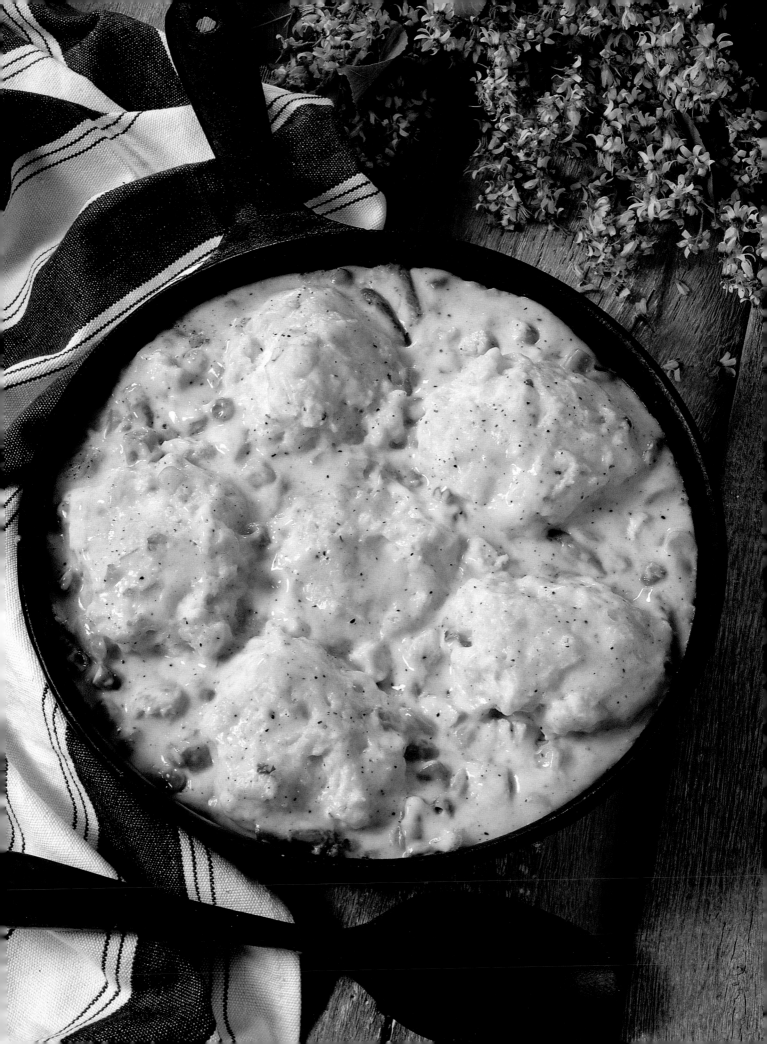

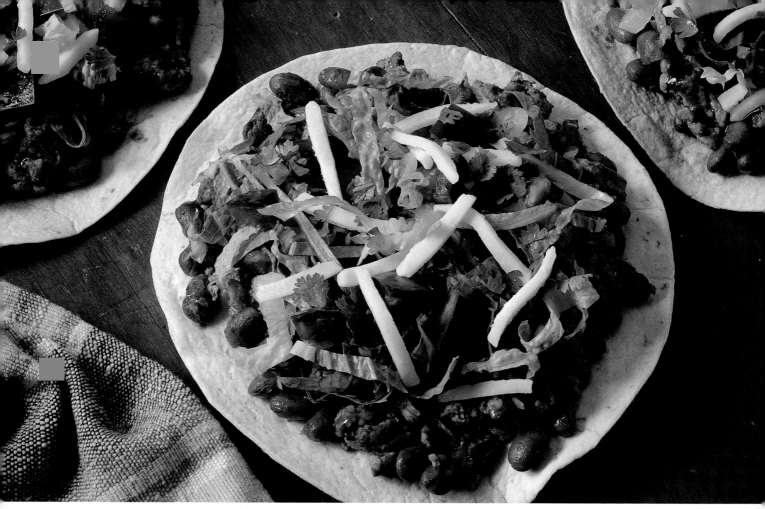

Turkey and Bean Tostadas

Turkey and Bean Tostadas

Quick Recipe   *(Pictured above)*

6 flour tortillas (8 inches)
1 pound 93% lean ground turkey
1 can (15 ounces) chili beans in chili
**   sauce**
1/2 teaspoon chili powder
3 cups shredded washed romaine lettuce
1 large tomato, chopped
1/4 cup chopped fresh cilantro
1/4 cup (1 ounce) shredded reduced-fat
**   Monterey Jack cheese**
1/2 cup low-fat sour cream (optional)

1. Preheat oven to 350°F. Place tortillas on baking sheets. Bake 7 minutes or until crisp. Place on individual plates.

2. Heat large nonstick skillet over medium-high heat until hot. Add turkey. Cook and stir until turkey is browned; drain.

3. Add beans and chili powder to skillet. Cook 5 minutes over medium heat.

4. Divide turkey mixture evenly among tortillas. Top with remaining ingredients and sour cream, if desired.   *Makes 6 servings*

Nutrients per Serving: 1 Tostada with toppings

Calories 288	**Fiber** 2g
Fat 10g (sat 2g)	**Cholesterol** 30mg
Protein 19g	**Sodium** 494mg
Carbohydrate 34g	

Exchanges: 2 starch, 1 vegetable, 2 lean meat

Thai Chicken Stir-Fry with Peanut Sauce

Quick Recipe

Peanut Sauce (recipe follows)
3/4 pound boneless skinless chicken breasts
Nonstick cooking spray
1 small onion, thinly sliced
2 tablespoons water
1 large red bell pepper, diced
1 package (10 ounces) fresh spinach leaves, washed and torn
2 cups hot cooked white rice
3 tablespoons chopped fresh basil, mint or cilantro leaves

1. Prepare Peanut Sauce; set aside. Slice chicken crosswise into thin strips. Spray large nonstick skillet with cooking spray; heat over high heat. Add chicken; stir-fry 4 minutes or until no longer pink in center. Remove chicken; set aside. Add onion and water to skillet; stir-fry 4 to 5 minutes or until water cooks away and onion is crisp-tender and golden. Stir in Peanut Sauce. Add bell pepper and chicken; bring to a boil. Cook and stir until slightly thickened and heated through.

2. Meanwhile, place spinach in another nonstick skillet. Cook and stir until spinach begins to wilt. Divide rice evenly among 4 plates. Place spinach over top. Spoon chicken mixture over spinach. Sprinkle with basil.

Makes 4 servings

Peanut Sauce

1/4 cup reduced-fat creamy peanut butter
1 tablespoon brown sugar
2 teaspoons dark sesame oil
1/4 teaspoon paprika
1/4 teaspoon coconut extract (optional)
1/2 cup fat-free reduced-sodium chicken broth
2 tablespoons reduced-sodium soy sauce
3 tablespoons lime juice

Stir together peanut butter, sugar, sesame oil, paprika and coconut extract, if desired, in small bowl until blended. Add chicken broth, soy sauce and lime juice; stir until smooth.

Makes about 1 cup

Nutrients per Serving: 1/2 cup cooked rice with about 1/2 cup steamed spinach and 1/2 cup Chicken mixture

Calories 381	Fiber 3g
Fat 11g (sat 2g)	Cholesterol 52mg
Protein 30g	Sodium 385mg
Carbohydrate 43g	

Exchanges: 2 starch, 2-1/2 vegetable, 3 lean meat

৵ ৵ ৵

Southern Breaded Catfish

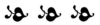

Quick Recipe

1/3 cup pecan halves, finely chopped
1/4 cup cornmeal
2 tablespoons all-purpose flour
1 teaspoon paprika
1/4 teaspoon ground red pepper
2 egg whites
4 catfish fillets (about 4 ounces each)
Nonstick cooking spray
4 cups hot cooked rice

1. Combine pecans, cornmeal, flour, paprika and ground red pepper in shallow bowl. Beat egg whites in small bowl with wire whisk until foamy. Dip catfish fillets in pecan mixture, then in egg whites and again in any remaining pecan mixture. Place fillets on plate; cover and refrigerate at least 15 minutes.

2. Spray large nonstick skillet with cooking spray; heat over medium-high heat. Place catfish fillets in single layer in skillet. Cook fillets 2 minutes per side or until golden brown and fillets flake easily when tested with fork. Serve over rice. Serve with vegetables and garnish, if desired.   *Makes 4 servings*

Nutrients per Serving: 1 fillet with 1 cup cooked white rice (without vegetables)

Calories 297	Fiber 2g
Fat 8g (sat 1g)	Cholesterol 65mg
Protein 22g	Sodium 76mg
Carbohydrate 33g	

Exchanges: 2 starch, 2-1/2 lean meat

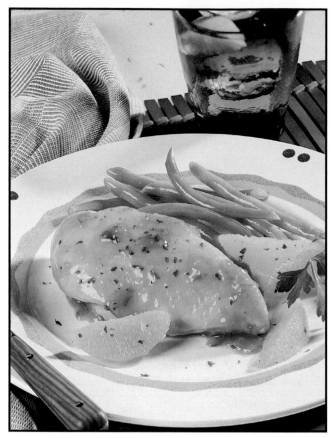

Quick Orange Chicken

2. Add chicken, coating both sides with sauce. Arrange chicken around edge of dish without overlapping. Cover with vented plastic wrap. Microwave at HIGH 3 minutes; turn chicken over. Microwave at MEDIUM-HIGH (70% power) 4 minutes or until chicken is no longer pink in center.

3. Remove chicken to serving plate. Microwave remaining sauce at HIGH 2 to 3 minutes or until slightly thickened.

4. To serve, spoon sauce over chicken; top with orange sections and parsley.

Makes 4 servings

Note: This recipe was tested in an 1100-watt microwave oven.

Nutrients per Serving: 1/4 of total recipe (1 Chicken breast per serving)

Calories 157	**Fiber** 1g
Fat 1g (sat <1g)	**Cholesterol** 66mg
Protein 27g	**Sodium** 234mg
Carbohydrate 8g	

Exchanges: 3 lean meat

Quick Orange Chicken

Quick Recipe   *(Pictured above)*

> 2 tablespoons frozen orange juice concentrate
> 1 tablespoon no-sugar-added orange marmalade
> 1 teaspoon Dijon mustard
> 1/4 teaspoon salt
> 4 boneless skinless chicken breasts (about 1 pound)
> 1/2 cup fresh orange sections
> 2 tablespoons chopped fresh parsley

Microwave Directions

1. For sauce, combine orange juice concentrate, marmalade, mustard and salt in 8-inch shallow round microwavable dish until juice concentrate is thawed.

Tip

Remember to follow these simple food safety tips for storing, handling and preparing chicken:

• Store raw poultry packages on the lowest shelf and away from other foods in the refrigerator.

• Thoroughly wash your hands and any cutting boards and utensils that come in contact with uncooked chicken with hot soapy water.

• Always cook chicken completely. Do not partially cook it and then store it to finish cooking later.

• Cook to an internal temperature of 170°F for white meat and 180°F for dark meat or until juices run clear.

Saucy Tomato-Pork Skillet

Quick Recipe   *(Pictured below)*

- 1 cup uncooked instant white rice
- 1 tablespoon cornstarch
- 2/3 cup reduced-sodium or regular tomato juice
- 2 tablespoons reduced-sodium or regular soy sauce
- 1/4 teaspoon paprika
- 3 boneless pork chops, cut 3/4 inch thick (about 3/4 pound)
- 1/4 teaspoon garlic salt
- 1/8 teaspoon red pepper flakes
- 2 slices uncooked bacon, chopped
- 3 medium tomatoes, chopped
- 2 green onions with tops, sliced diagonally

1. Prepare rice according to package directions; set aside.

2. Combine cornstarch, tomato juice, soy sauce and paprika in small bowl, stirring until cornstarch dissolves. Set aside.

3. Slice pork across the grain into 1/4-inch slices; place in medium bowl. Sprinkle pork with garlic salt and red pepper flakes; mix well.

4. Cook bacon in medium skillet over medium heat. Remove bacon from skillet using slotted spoon; set aside. Add pork, tomatoes and green onions to skillet; cook over medium-high heat 3 minutes or until pork is barely pink in center. Stir in reserved tomato juice mixture; cook, stirring constantly, 1 minute or until sauce thickens slightly. Remove from heat; stir in bacon.

5. Serve pork mixture over rice.

Makes 4 servings

Nutrients per Serving: 1-1/2 cups Pork mixture with 1/2 cup cooked rice

Calories 307	**Fiber** 1g
Fat 10g (sat 4g)	**Cholesterol** 62mg
Protein 23g	**Sodium** 492mg
Carbohydrate 26g	

Exchanges: 1-1/2 starch, 1 vegetable, 2 lean meat, 1 fat

Saucy Tomato-Pork Skillet

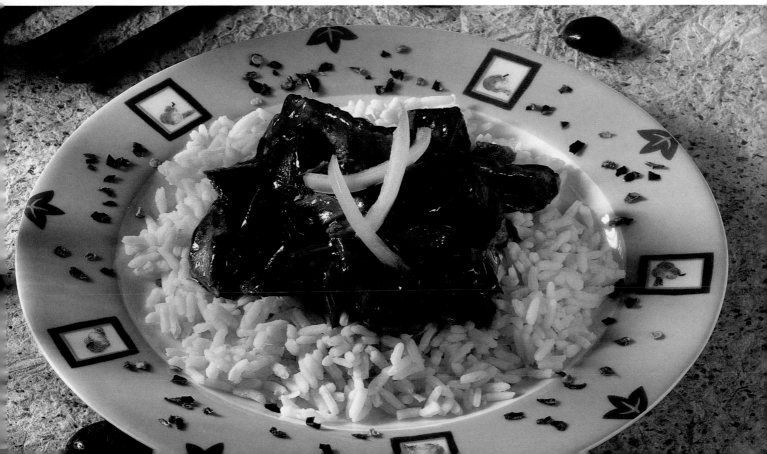

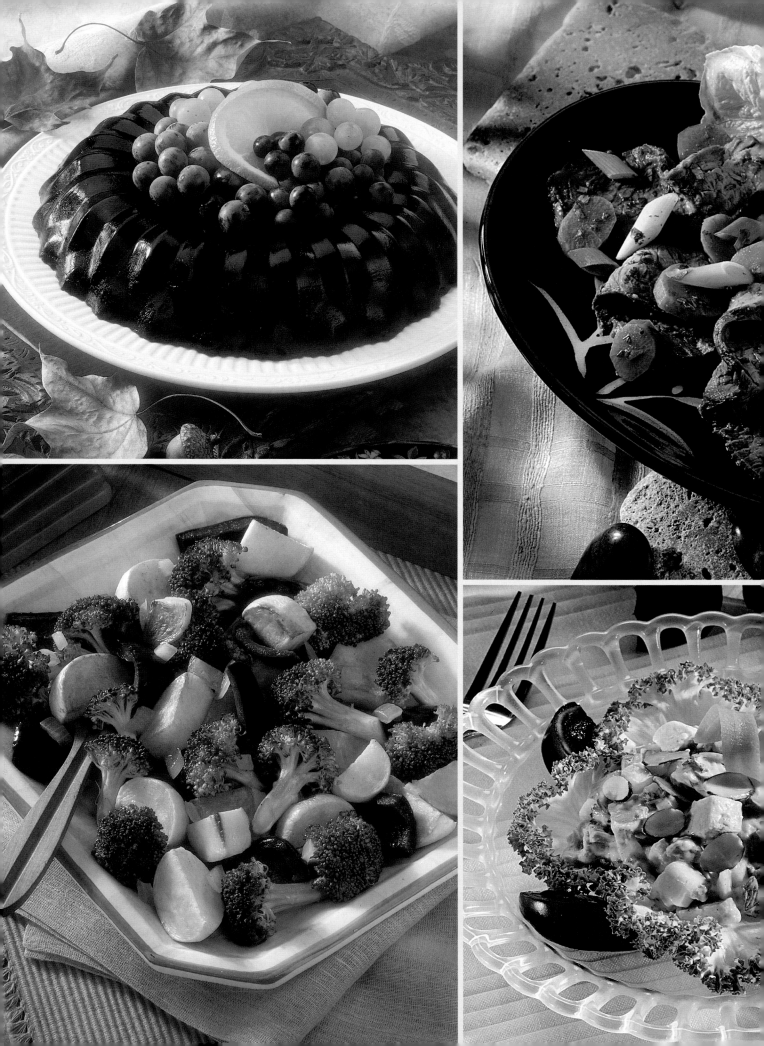

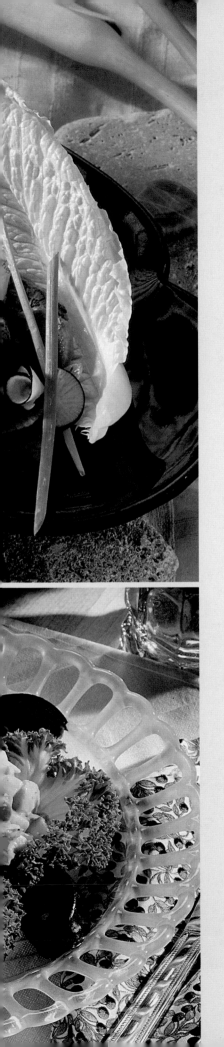

Sides & Salads

❧ ❧ ❧

Cranberry Fruit Mold

(Pictured at left)

2 cups boiling water

1 package (8-serving size) *or* 2 packages (4-serving size) JELL-O® Brand Cranberry Flavor Gelatin Dessert *or* JELL-O® Brand Cranberry Flavor Sugar Free Low Calorie Gelatin Dessert

1-1/2 cups cold juice, ginger ale, lemon-lime carbonated beverage, seltzer or water

2 cups halved green and/or red seedless grapes

1 can (11 ounces) mandarin orange segments, drained

STIR boiling water into gelatin in large bowl at least 2 minutes until completely dissolved. Stir in cold juice. Refrigerate about 1-1/2 hours or until thickened (spoon drawn through leaves definite impression). Stir in fruit. Spoon into 6-cup mold.

REFRIGERATE 4 hours or until firm. Unmold. Garnish as desired.

Makes 10 servings

Nutrients per Serving: 1/10 of total recipe (using JELL-O® Brand Cranberry Flavor Sugar Free Low Calorie Gelatin Dessert and seltzer)

Calories 60	**Fiber** 1g
Fat <1g (sat <1g)	**Cholesterol** 0mg
Protein 1g	**Sodium** 47mg
Carbohydrate 13g	

Exchanges: 1 fruit

Clockwise from top left: Cranberry Fruit Mold, Thai Beef Salad (page 117), Light Chicken Vegetable Salad (page 114) and Roasted Fall Vegetables (page 118)

Indian-Style Vegetable Stir-Fry

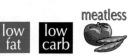

Quick Recipe   *(Pictured at right)*

- 1 teaspoon canola oil
- 1 teaspoon curry powder
- 1 teaspoon ground cumin
- 1/8 teaspoon red pepper flakes
- 1-1/2 teaspoons minced seeded jalapeño pepper*
- 2 cloves garlic, minced
- 3/4 cup chopped red bell pepper
- 3/4 cup thinly sliced carrots
- 3 cups cauliflower florets
- 1/2 cup water, divided
- 1/2 teaspoon salt
- 2 teaspoons finely chopped fresh cilantro (optional)

*Jalapeño peppers can sting and irritate the skin; wear rubber gloves when handling peppers and do not touch eyes. Wash hands after handling peppers.

1. Heat oil in large nonstick skillet over medium-high heat. Add curry powder, cumin and red pepper flakes; cook and stir about 30 seconds.

2. Stir in jalapeño pepper and garlic. Add bell pepper and carrots; mix well. Add cauliflower; reduce heat to medium.

3. Stir in 1/4 cup water; cook and stir until water evaporates. Add remaining 1/4 cup water; cover and cook about 8 to 10 minutes or until vegetables are crisp-tender, stirring occasionally.

4. Add salt; mix well. Sprinkle with cilantro and garnish with mizuna and additional red bell pepper, if desired.   *Makes 6 servings*

Nutrients per Serving: 1 cup Stir-Fry

Calories 40	**Fiber** 2g
Fat 1g (sat <1g)	**Cholesterol** 0mg
Protein 2g	**Sodium** 198mg
Carbohydrate 7g	

Exchanges: 1-1/2 vegetable

Herbed Green Beans

Quick Recipe

- 1 pound fresh green beans, stem ends removed
- 1 teaspoon extra-virgin olive oil
- 2 tablespoons chopped fresh basil *or* 2 teaspoons dried basil leaves

1. Steam green beans 5 minutes or until crisp-tender. Rinse under cold running water; drain and set aside.

2. Just before serving, heat oil over medium-low heat in large nonstick skillet. Add basil; cook and stir 1 minute, then add green beans. Cook until heated through.

3. Garnish with additional fresh basil, if desired. Serve immediately.   *Makes 6 servings*

Nutrients per Serving: 2/3 cup

Calories 26	**Fiber** 0g
Fat 1g (sat <1g)	**Cholesterol** 0mg
Protein 1g	**Sodium** 10mg
Carbohydrate 5g	

Exchanges: 1 vegetable

Tip

When buying green beans, look for vivid green, crisp beans without scars. Pods should be well shaped and slim with small seeds. Buy beans of uniform size to ensure even cooking, and avoid bruised or large beans.

Indian-Style Vegetable Stir-Fry

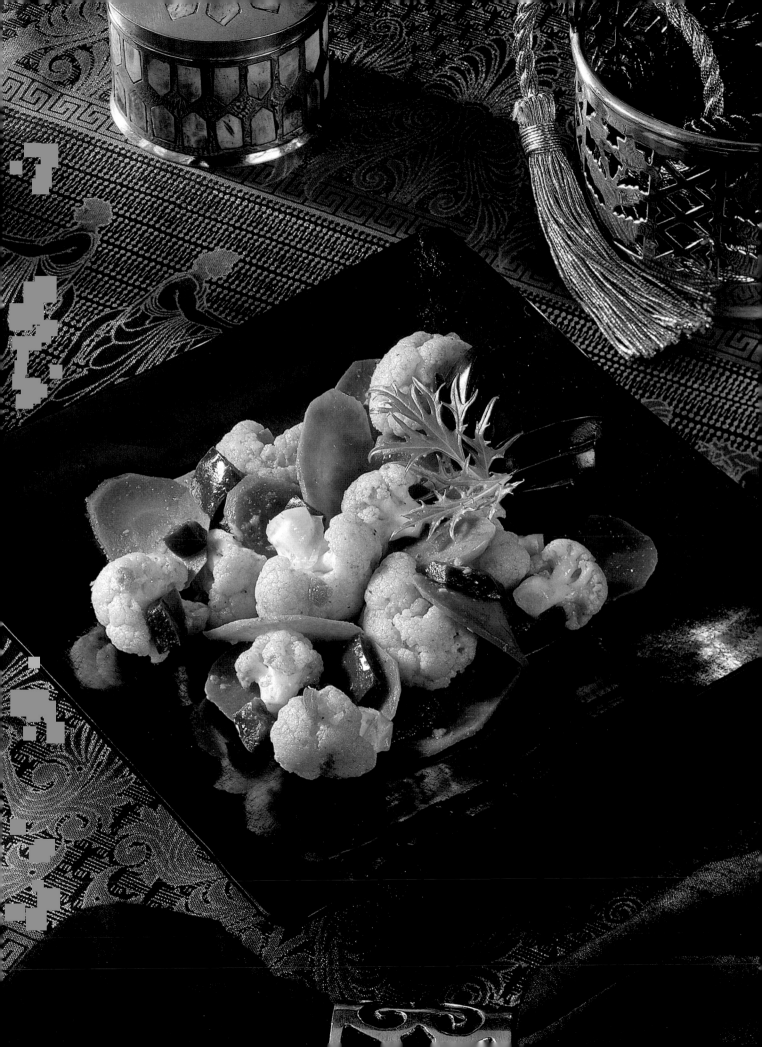

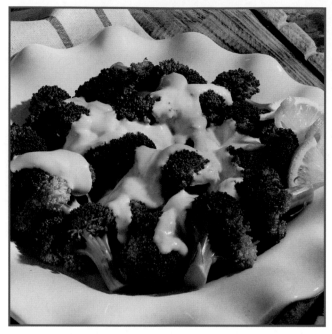

Broccoli with Creamy Lemon Sauce

Broccoli with Creamy Lemon Sauce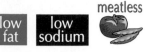

Quick Recipe   *(Pictured above)*

2 tablespoons fat-free mayonnaise
4-1/2 teaspoons reduced-fat sour cream
1 tablespoon fat-free milk
1 to 1-1/2 teaspoons lemon juice
1/8 teaspoon ground turmeric
1-1/4 cups hot cooked broccoli florets

1. Combine all ingredients except broccoli in top of double boiler. Cook over simmering water 5 minutes or until heated through, stirring constantly.

2. Serve sauce over hot cooked broccoli.

Makes 2 servings

Nutrients per Serving: 1/2 of total recipe

Calories 44	**Fiber** 2g
Fat 1g (sat <1g)	**Cholesterol** 4mg
Protein 2g	**Sodium** 216mg
Carbohydrate 7g	

Exchanges: 2 vegetable

Santa Fe Grilled Vegetable Salad

Quick Recipe

2 baby eggplants (6 ounces each), halved
1 medium yellow summer squash, halved
1 medium zucchini, halved
1 medium green bell pepper, cored and quartered
1 medium red bell pepper, cored and quartered
1 small onion, peeled and halved
1/2 cup orange juice
2 tablespoons lime juice
1 tablespoon olive oil
2 cloves garlic, minced
1 teaspoon dried oregano leaves
1/4 teaspoon *each* salt, ground red pepper and black pepper
2 tablespoons chopped fresh cilantro or parsley

1. Combine vegetables in large bowl. Combine all remaining ingredients except cilantro in small bowl; mix well. Pour marinade over vegetables; toss to coat.

2. Spray grid with nonstick cooking spray. Prepare coals for direct grilling. Place vegetables on grill, 2 to 3 inches from hot coals; reserve marinade. Grill 3 to 4 minutes per side or until tender and lightly charred; cool 10 minutes. (Or, place vegetables on rack of broiler pan coated with nonstick cooking spray; reserve marinade. Broil 2 to 3 inches from heat, 3 to 4 minutes per side or until tender; cool 10 minutes.)

3. Remove peel from eggplant, if desired. Slice vegetables into bite-size pieces; return to marinade. Stir in cilantro; toss to coat.

Makes 8 servings

Nutrients per Serving: 1 cup Salad

Calories 63	**Fiber** 2g
Fat 2g (sat <1g)	**Cholesterol** <1mg
Protein 2g	**Sodium** 70mg
Carbohydrate 11g	

Exchanges: 2 vegetable, 1/2 fat

Vegetable Confetti Rice

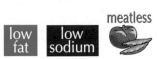 low fat | low sodium | meatless

- 1 tablespoon olive oil
- 1 cup finely chopped celery
- 1/2 cup uncooked long-grain white rice
- 1/2 cup bottled roasted sweet red peppers, diced
- 1 can (14-1/2 ounces) fat-free reduced-sodium chicken broth
- 2 bags (10 ounces each) mixed broccoli-cauliflower florets, cut into equal-size pieces

1. Heat oil in large nonstick skillet over medium heat. Add celery and sauté, stirring occasionally, until crisp-tender, about 5 to 6 minutes.

2. Add rice to skillet; sauté, stirring, until rice becomes opaque, about 3 to 4 minutes. Add diced red peppers and stir. Add broth; cover tightly with lid and cook until rice is just cooked through, about 12 minutes.

3. Add broccoli-cauliflower florets to skillet; cover tightly and cook until vegetables are tender, about 10 minutes. Add water by tablespoonful, if necessary. Stir vegetables and rice together gently with spatula before serving.

Makes 8 servings

Nutrients per Serving: 1/2 cup Vegetable Confetti Rice

Calories 90	**Fiber** 2g
Fat 2g (sat <1g)	**Cholesterol** 5mg
Protein 3g	**Sodium** 103mg
Carbohydrate 14g	

Exchanges: 1/2 starch, 1 vegetable, 1/2 fat

Tip

To cut a bell pepper into strips, stand the pepper on its end on a cutting board. Cut off 3 to 4 lengthwise slices from the sides, cutting close to, but not through, the stem. Discard the stem and seeds. Scrape out any remaining seeds, and rinse the inside of the pepper under cold running water. Slice each piece lengthwise into strips.

Green Chili Vegetable Salad

low fat | meatless

Quick Recipe   (Pictured below)

- 4 cups torn romaine lettuce leaves
- 1 large green bell pepper, cut into strips
- 1 cup halved cherry tomatoes
- 3 tablespoons shredded reduced-fat colby or Cheddar cheese
- 1/4 cup fat-free mayonnaise or salad dressing
- 2 tablespoons plain reduced-fat yogurt
- 1 can (4 ounces) diced green chilies, drained
- 1/4 teaspoon ground cumin

1. Combine lettuce, bell pepper, tomatoes and cheese in large bowl. Combine mayonnaise, yogurt, green chilies and cumin in small bowl.

2. Add dressing to salad; toss to combine.

Makes 4 servings

Nutrients per Serving: about 1-3/4 cups Salad

Calories 81	**Fiber** 4g
Fat 2g (sat 1g)	**Cholesterol** 4mg
Protein 4g	**Sodium** 168mg
Carbohydrate 14g	

Exchanges: 3 vegetable

Green Chili Vegetable Salad

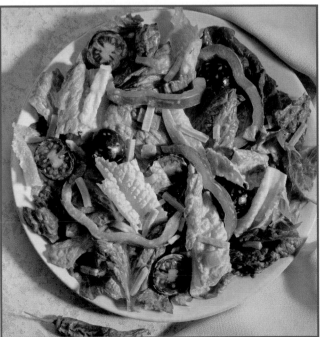

Garlic Lovers' Chicken Caesar Salad

Quick Recipe   (Pictured at right)

DRESSING

1 can (10-3/4 ounces) reduced-fat condensed cream of chicken soup, undiluted

1/2 cup fat-free reduced-sodium chicken broth

1/4 cup balsamic vinegar or red wine vinegar

1/4 cup fat-free shredded Parmesan cheese, divided

3 cloves garlic, minced

1 tablespoon Worcestershire sauce

1/4 teaspoon black pepper

SALAD

2 heads romaine lettuce (12 ounces each), torn into 2-inch pieces

4 grilled boneless skinless chicken breasts (about 1 pound), cut into 2-inch strips

1/2 cup fat-free herb-seasoned croutons

1. Combine soup, chicken broth, vinegar, 2 tablespoons Parmesan cheese, garlic, Worcestershire sauce and pepper in food processor or blender; process until smooth.

2. Combine lettuce and 1 cup dressing in large salad bowl; toss well to coat. Top with chicken and croutons; sprinkle with remaining 2 tablespoons cheese.   *Makes 8 servings*

Nutrients per Serving: 1-1/4 cups lettuce mixture with about 4 (2-inch) chicken strips, 1 tablespoon croutons and 3/4 teaspoon sprinkled cheese

Calories 132	**Fiber** 1g
Fat 2g (sat 1g)	**Cholesterol** 40mg
Protein 17g	**Sodium** 202mg
Carbohydrate 10g	

Exchanges: 1/2 starch, 2 lean meat

Lemon Broccoli Pasta

Quick Recipe

Nonstick cooking spray

3 tablespoons sliced green onions

1 clove garlic, minced

2 cups fat-free reduced-sodium chicken broth

1-1/2 teaspoons grated lemon peel

1/8 teaspoon black pepper

2 cups fresh or frozen broccoli florets

3 ounces uncooked angel hair pasta

1/3 cup reduced-fat sour cream

2 tablespoons grated reduced-fat Parmesan cheese

1. Generously spray large nonstick saucepan with cooking spray; heat over medium heat until hot. Add green onions and garlic; cook and stir 3 minutes or until onions are tender.

2. Stir chicken broth, lemon peel and pepper into saucepan; bring to a boil over high heat. Stir in broccoli and pasta; return to a boil.

3. Reduce heat to low. Simmer, uncovered, 6 to 7 minutes or until pasta is tender, stirring frequently.

4. Remove saucepan from heat. Stir in sour cream until well blended. Let stand 5 minutes. Top with cheese before serving. Garnish as desired.   *Makes 6 servings*

Nutrients per Serving: 1 cup Lemon Broccoli Pasta

Calories 100	**Fiber** 3g
Fat 2g (sat <1g)	**Cholesterol** 6mg
Protein 7g	**Sodium** 176mg
Carbohydrate 14g	

Exchanges: 1/2 starch, 1-1/2 vegetable, 1/2 fat

Garlic Lovers' Chicken Caesar Salad

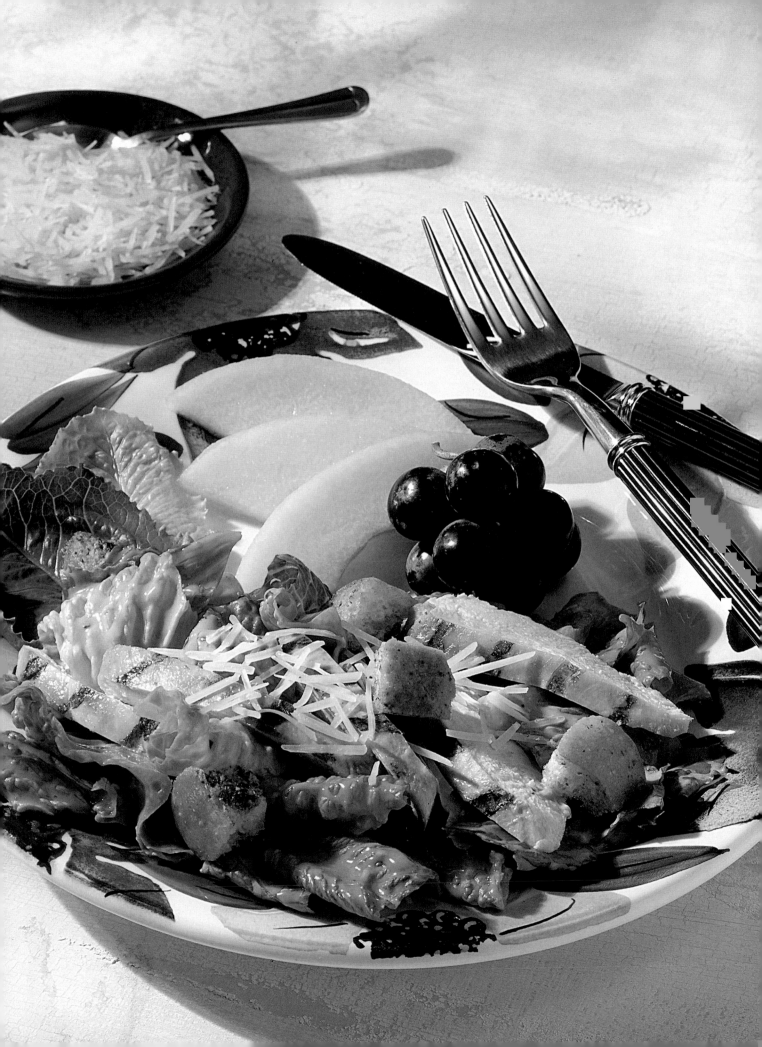

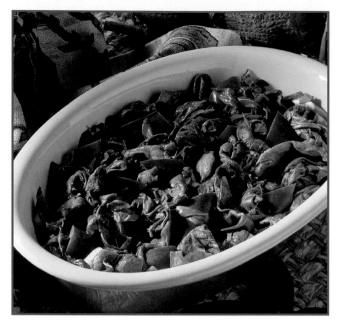

Hot and Spicy Spinach

Hot and Spicy Spinach

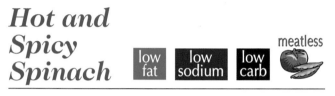

low fat | low sodium | low carb | meatless

Quick Recipe   *(Pictured above)*

Nonstick cooking spray
1 medium red bell pepper, cut into 1-inch pieces
1 clove garlic, minced
1 pound prewashed fresh spinach, rinsed, drained and chopped
1 tablespoon prepared mustard
1 teaspoon lemon juice
1/4 teaspoon red pepper flakes

1. Spray large nonstick skillet with cooking spray; heat over medium heat. Add bell pepper and garlic; cook and stir 3 minutes. Add spinach; cook and stir 3 minutes or just until spinach begins to wilt.

2. Stir in mustard, lemon juice and red pepper flakes. Serve immediately.   *Makes 4 servings*

Nutrients per Serving: 1 cup Spinach

Calories 37	**Fiber** 3g
Fat 1g (sat <1g)	**Cholesterol** 0mg
Protein 4g	**Sodium** 138mg
Carbohydrate 6g	

Exchanges: 1-1/2 vegetable

Light Chicken Vegetable Salad

low carb

(Pictured on page 106)

1-1/4 pounds skinless chicken breasts, cooked and cut into 3/4-inch pieces
1/3 cup chopped zucchini
1/3 cup chopped carrot
2 tablespoons chopped onion
2 tablespoons chopped fresh parsley
1/3 cup fat-free mayonnaise
1/4 cup fat-free sour cream
1/4 teaspoon salt
1/8 teaspoon black pepper
Kale or lettuce leaves (optional)
3 medium tomatoes, cut into wedges
1/4 cup toasted sliced almonds

1. Combine chicken, zucchini, carrot, onion and parsley in large bowl.

2. Combine mayonnaise, sour cream, salt and pepper in small bowl. Add to chicken mixture; mix well. Cover and refrigerate at least 2 hours.

3. Line 6 plates with kale leaves, if desired. Divided salad evenly among plates. Surround with tomato wedges; sprinkle evenly with almonds. Garnish, if desired.

Makes 6 servings

Nutrients per Serving: about 3/4 cup Salad with 1/2 of a tomato and 2 teaspoons almonds

Calories 178	**Fiber** 2g
Fat 4g (sat 1g)	**Cholesterol** 55mg
Protein 24g	**Sodium** 274mg
Carbohydrate 9g	

Exchanges: 1 vegetable, 3 lean meat

Three-Pepper Tuna Salad

Quick Recipe   (Pictured at bottom right)

 3/4 cup water
 2 cups thinly sliced zucchini
 1/2 cup red bell pepper strips
 1/2 cup green bell pepper strips
 1/2 cup yellow bell pepper strips
 1 cup cherry tomatoes, halved
 1 can (6 ounces) solid albacore tuna packed in water, drained and flaked
 1/4 cup chopped green onions with tops
 1/4 cup chopped fresh basil
 2-1/2 tablespoons red wine vinegar or cider vinegar
 1 tablespoon olive oil
 1/2 teaspoon minced fresh garlic
 1/2 teaspoon fresh marjoram
 1/8 teaspoon black pepper

1. Combine water, zucchini and bell pepper strips in medium saucepan. Steam vegetables about 10 minutes or until crisp-tender. Remove from heat; drain any excess water. Transfer to serving bowl. Add tomatoes, tuna, green onions and basil.

2. Combine vinegar, oil, garlic, marjoram and black pepper in jar or bottle with tight-fitting lid; shake well. Pour dressing over vegetable mixture; mix well. Garnish as desired.

Makes 4 servings

Nutrients per Serving: about 1-1/3 cups Salad

Calories 134	**Fiber** 3g
Fat 5g (sat 1g)	**Cholesterol** 18mg
Protein 14g	**Sodium** 175mg
Carbohydrate 11g	

Exchanges: 2 vegetable, 1-1/2 lean meat

Collard Greens

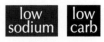

 4 bunches collards, stems removed and leaves washed very well and torn into bite-size pieces
 2 cups water
 1/4 cup olive oil
 1/4 teaspoon salt
 1/4 teaspoon black pepper
 1/2 medium red bell pepper, cored, seeded and cut into strips
 1/3 medium green bell pepper, cored, seeded and cut into strips

1. Place 1/2 of collards in large saucepan. Add all remaining ingredients. Bring to a boil. Add remaining collards after first bunch begins to wilt.

2. Reduce heat and simmer about 1 to 1-1/2 hours or until tender.

Makes 10 servings

Nutrients per Serving: 1/2 cup

Calories 64	**Fiber** 2g
Fat 5g (sat <1g)	**Cholesterol** 0mg
Protein 3g	**Sodium** 14mg
Carbohydrate 6g	

Exchanges: 1 vegetable, 1 fat

Three-Pepper Tuna Salad

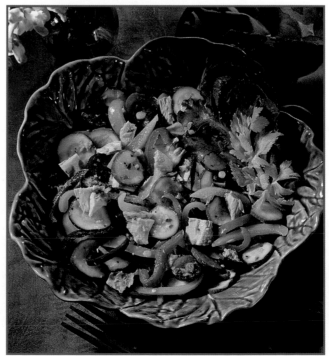

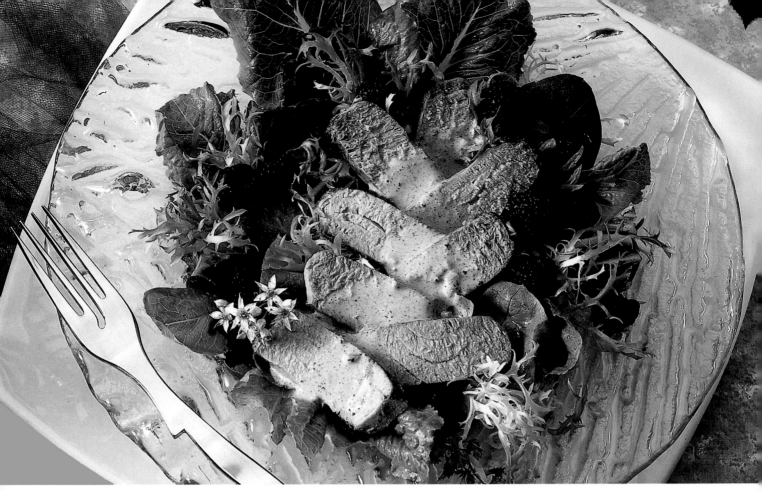

Broiled Tuna and Raspberry Salad

Broiled Tuna and Raspberry Salad

high fiber

cooking for 1 or 2

Quick Recipe   *(Pictured above)*

1/2 cup fat-free ranch salad dressing

1/4 cup raspberry vinegar or red wine vinegar

1-1/2 teaspoons Cajun seasoning

1 thick-sliced tuna steak (about 6 to 8 ounces)

2 cups torn romaine lettuce leaves

1 cup torn mixed baby lettuce leaves

1/2 cup fresh raspberries

1. Combine salad dressing, vinegar and Cajun seasoning in large glass measuring cup. Pour 1/4 cup salad dressing mixture into resealable plastic food storage bag to use as marinade, reserving remaining mixture. Add tuna to marinade. Seal bag; turn to coat tuna. Marinate in the refrigerator 10 minutes, turning once.

2. Preheat broiler. Spray rack of broiler pan with nonstick cooking spray. Place tuna on rack. Broil tuna 4 inches from heat 5 minutes. Turn tuna and brush with marinade; discard remaining marinade. Broil 5 minutes more or until tuna flakes in center when tested with fork. Cool 5 minutes. Cut into 1/4-inch-thick slices.

3. Toss lettuces together in large bowl; divide evenly between two serving plates. Top evenly with tuna and raspberries; drizzle with reserved salad dressing mixture.   *Makes 2 servings*

Nutrients per Serving: 1/2 of total recipe

Calories 215	**Fiber** 5g
Fat 5g (sat 1g)	**Cholesterol** 35mg
Protein 24g	**Sodium** 427mg
Carbohydrate 18g	

Exchanges: 1/2 fruit, 1 vegetable, 3 lean meat

Thai Beef Salad

(Pictured on page 106)

8 ounces beef flank steak

1/4 cup reduced-sodium soy sauce

2 jalapeño peppers,* finely chopped

2 tablespoons packed brown sugar

1 clove garlic, minced

1/2 cup lime juice

6 green onions, thinly sliced

4 carrots, diagonally cut into thin slices

1/2 cup finely chopped fresh cilantro

4 romaine lettuce leaves

Jalapeño peppers can sting and irritate the skin; wear rubber gloves when handling peppers and do not touch eyes. Wash hands after handling peppers.

1. Place flank steak in large resealable plastic food storage bag. Combine soy sauce, jalapeños, brown sugar and garlic in small bowl; mix well. Pour mixture over flank steak.

2. Close bag securely; turn to coat steak. Marinate in refrigerator 2 hours.

3. Preheat broiler. Drain steak; discard marinade. Place steak on rack of broiler pan. Broil 4 inches from heat about 4 minutes per side or until desired doneness. Remove from heat; let stand 15 minutes.

4. Thinly slice steak across grain. Toss with lime juice, green onions, carrots and cilantro in large bowl.

5. Serve salad immediately on lettuce leaves. Garnish with chives and radish flowers, if desired. *Makes 4 servings*

Nutrients per Serving: 1 cup Salad with 1 lettuce leaf

Calories 141	**Fiber** 3g
Fat 4g (sat 2g)	**Cholesterol** 27mg
Protein 13g	**Sodium** 238mg
Carbohydrate 14g	

Exchanges: 2-1/2 vegetable, 1-1/2 lean meat

Savory Green Bean Casserole

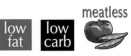

2 teaspoons CRISCO® Oil*

1 medium onion, chopped

1/2 medium green bell pepper, chopped

1 package (10 ounces) frozen green beans, thawed

1 can (8 ounces) tomatoes, drained

2 tablespoons nonfat mayonnaise dressing

1/4 teaspoon salt

1/8 teaspoon crushed red pepper

1/8 teaspoon garlic powder

1/4 cup plain dry bread crumbs

Use your favorite Crisco Oil product.

1. Heat oven to 375°F. Oil 1-quart casserole lightly. Place cooling rack on countertop.

2. Heat 2 teaspoons oil in large skillet on medium heat. Add onion and green pepper. Cook and stir until tender.

3. Add beans, tomatoes, mayonnaise dressing, salt, red pepper and garlic powder. Heat thoroughly, stirring occasionally.

4. Spoon into casserole. Sprinkle with bread crumbs. Bake at 375°F for 30 minutes. *Do not overbake.* Remove casserole to cooling rack. Serve warm. *Makes 8 servings*

Nutrients per Serving: 1/2 cup Casserole

Calories 51	**Fiber** 2g
Fat 1g (sat <1g)	**Cholesterol** 0mg
Protein 1g	**Sodium** 179mg
Carbohydrate 8g	

Exchanges: 2 vegetable

Eggplant Squash Bake

high fiber · meatless

(Pictured at right)

- 1/2 cup chopped onion
- 1 clove garlic, minced
  Olive oil-flavored nonstick cooking spray
- 1 cup part-skim ricotta cheese
- 1 jar (4 ounces) diced pimientos, drained
- 1/4 cup grated Parmesan cheese
- 2 tablespoons fat-free milk
- 1-1/2 teaspoons dried marjoram leaves
- 3/4 teaspoon dried tarragon leaves
- 1/4 teaspoon salt
- 1/4 teaspoon ground nutmeg
- 1/4 teaspoon black pepper
- 1 cup no-sugar-added meatless spaghetti sauce, divided
- 1/2 pound eggplant, peeled and cut into thin crosswise slices
- 6 ounces zucchini, cut in half, then lengthwise into thin slices
- 6 ounces yellow summer squash, cut in half, then lengthwise into thin slices
- 2 tablespoons shredded part-skim mozzarella cheese

Microwave Directions

1. Combine onion and garlic in medium microwavable bowl. Spray lightly with cooking spray. Microwave at HIGH 1 minute. Add ricotta, pimientos, Parmesan, milk, marjoram, tarragon, salt, nutmeg and pepper.

2. Spray 9- or 10-inch round microwavable baking dish with cooking spray. Spread 1/3 cup spaghetti sauce in bottom of dish. Layer half of eggplant, zucchini and summer squash in dish; top with ricotta mixture. Layer remaining eggplant, zucchini and summer squash over ricotta mixture. Top with remaining 2/3 cup spaghetti sauce. Cover with vented plastic wrap. Microwave at HIGH 17 to 19 minutes or until vegetables are tender, rotating dish every 6 minutes. Top with mozzarella cheese. Let stand 10 minutes before serving.

Makes 4 servings

Note: This recipe was tested in an 1100-watt microwave oven.

Nutrients per Serving: 1 cup Eggplant Squash Bake

Calories 190	**Fiber** 5g
Fat 8g (sat 6g)	**Cholesterol** 25mg
Protein 13g	**Sodium** 647mg
Carbohydrate 19g	

Exchanges: 4 vegetable, 1 lean meat, 1 fat

Ǝ Ǝ Ǝ

Roasted Fall Vegetables

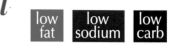

low fat · low sodium · low carb

(Pictured on page 106)

- 2 cups small broccoli florets
- 1 large red bell pepper, cut into squares
- 1 cup cubed turnip (1-inch cubes)
- 1/2 cup diced onion
- 1 tablespoon balsamic vinegar or red wine vinegar
- 2 teaspoons olive oil
- 1/2 cup fat-free reduced-sodium chicken broth or water
- 4 sprigs fresh thyme *or* 1/4 teaspoon dried thyme leaves
- 1/4 teaspoon salt
  Black pepper

Preheat oven to 425°F. Combine broccoli, bell pepper, turnip and onion in heavy shallow roasting pan. Whisk together vinegar and oil; pour over vegetables, tossing to coat. Pour chicken broth around vegetables. Add thyme sprigs. Roast vegetables about 30 minutes or until tender, stirring occasionally. Remove from oven. Season with salt and black pepper.

Makes 6 servings

Nutrients per Serving: 1/3 cup Roasted Fall Vegetables

Calories 36	**Fiber** 2g
Fat 2g (sat <1g)	**Cholesterol** 0mg
Protein 2g	**Sodium** 133mg
Carbohydrate 4g	

Exchanges: 1 vegetable, 1/2 fat

Eggplant Squash Bake

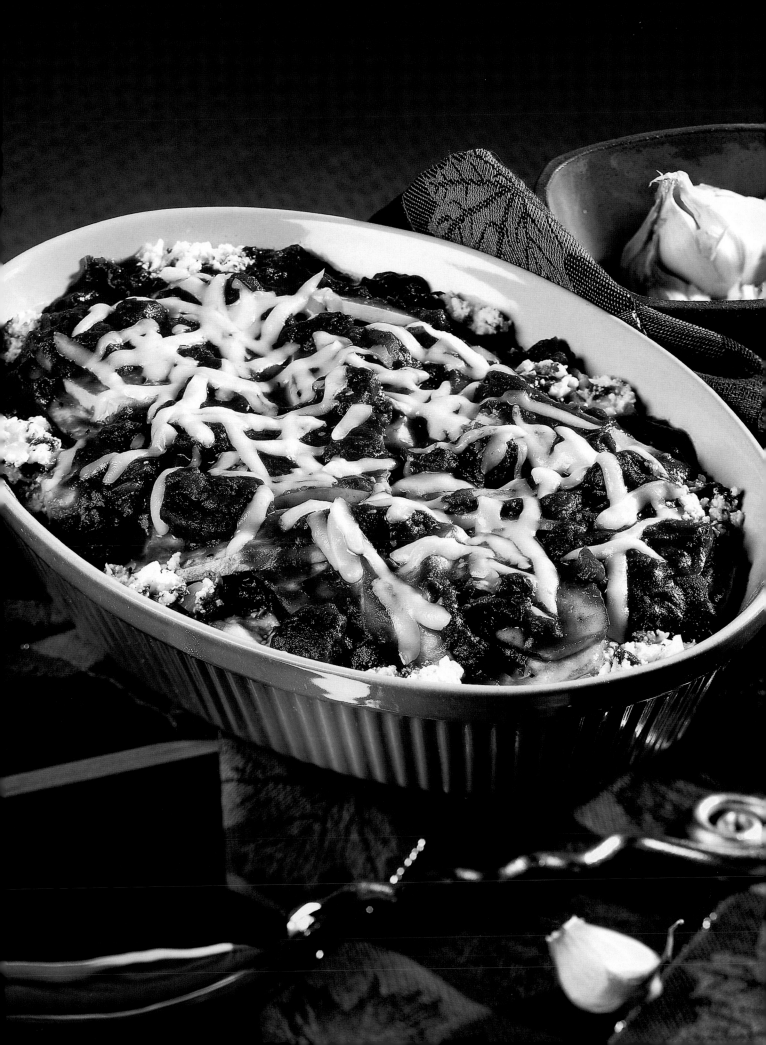

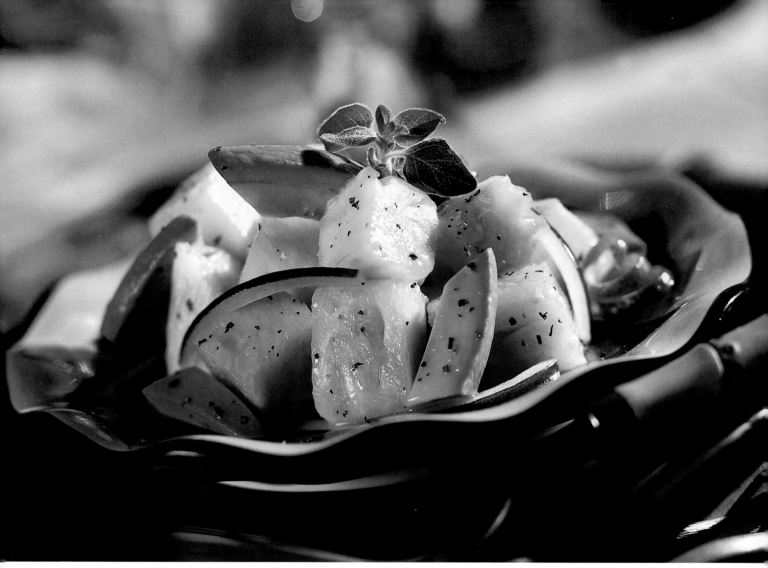

Pineapple Avocado Salad

Pineapple Avocado Salad 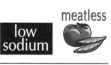 low sodium meatless

Quick Recipe   (Pictured above)

2 cups (1/2-inch pieces) fresh pineapple
3/4 cup sliced avocado
1/4 cup thinly sliced red onion
1 tablespoon finely chopped fresh
oregano
Freshly ground black pepper
3 tablespoons fresh lime juice
1 teaspoon peanut or safflower oil
2 packets NatraTaste® Brand Sugar
Substitute
1/8 teaspoon salt
1 garlic clove, minced

1. Place pineapple on a plate, and top with avocado, onion, oregano and pepper.

2. Combine remaining ingredients in a small jar with a lid. Shake, and using a spoon, drizzle dressing over salad.   *Makes 4 servings*

Nutrients per Serving: about 3/4 cup Salad with 1 tablespoon dressing

Calories 110	**Fiber** 2g
Fat 5g (sat <1g)	**Cholesterol** 0mg
Protein 1g	**Sodium** 80mg
Carbohydrate 15g	

Exchanges: 1 fruit, 1 fat

Cool and Creamy Pea Salad with Cucumbers and Red Onion

 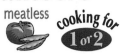

Quick Recipe

2 tablespoons finely chopped red onion
1 tablespoon reduced-fat mayonnaise
1/8 teaspoon salt
1/8 teaspoon black pepper
1/2 cup frozen green peas, thawed
1/4 cup diced red bell pepper
1/4 cup diced cucumber

1. Combine onion, mayonnaise, salt and black pepper in medium bowl; stir until well blended.

2. Add remaining ingredients and toss gently to coat. *Makes 2 servings*

Nutrients per Serving: 1/2 cup Salad

Calories 65	**Fiber** 3g
Fat 3g (sat 1g)	**Cholesterol** 3mg
Protein 2g	**Sodium** 238mg
Carbohydrate 8g	

Exchanges: 1-1/2 vegetable, 1/2 fat

❧ ❧ ❧

Pasta and Tuna Filled Peppers

(Pictured at right)

3/4 cup uncooked ditalini or other small pasta
4 medium green, red or yellow bell peppers
1 cup chopped seeded tomatoes
1 can (6 ounces) white tuna packed in water, drained and flaked
1/2 cup chopped celery
1/2 cup (2 ounces) shredded reduced-fat Cheddar cheese
1/4 cup fat-free mayonnaise or salad dressing
1 teaspoon salt-free garlic and herb seasoning
2 tablespoons shredded reduced-fat Cheddar cheese (optional)

Microwave Directions

1. Cook pasta according to package directions, omitting salt. Drain; rinse in cool water. Set aside.

2. Cut thin slice from top of each pepper. Remove veins and seeds from insides of peppers. Rinse; place peppers, cut sides down, on paper towels to drain.

3. Combine pasta, tomatoes, tuna, celery, 1/2 cup cheese, mayonnaise and seasoning in large bowl until well blended; spoon evenly into pepper shells.

4. Arrange peppers around outer edge of large microwave-safe plate; cover with waxed paper. Microwave at HIGH 8 to 10 minutes or until peppers are tender and pasta mixture is hot, turning halfway through cooking time. Top evenly with remaining 2 tablespoons cheese before serving, if desired. Garnish as desired. *Makes 4 servings*

Note: This recipe was tested in an 1100-watt microwave oven.

Nutrients per Serving: 1 Pepper filled with about 1 cup Pasta-Tuna mixture

Calories 216	**Fiber** 2g
Fat 4g (sat 1g)	**Cholesterol** 26mg
Protein 19g	**Sodium** 574mg
Carbohydrate 27g	

Exchanges: 1-1/2 starch, 1 vegetable, 1-1/2 lean meat

Pasta and Tuna Filled Pepper

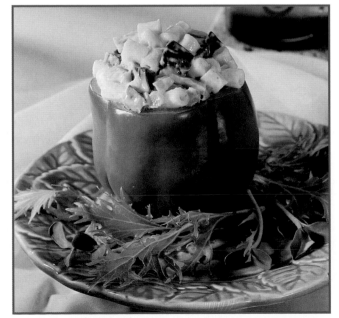

Hot Chinese Chicken Salad

Quick Recipe   *(Pictured at right)*

8 ounces fresh or steamed Chinese egg noodles or angel hair pasta

1/4 cup fat-free reduced-sodium chicken broth

2 tablespoons reduced-sodium soy sauce

2 tablespoons rice wine vinegar or white wine vinegar

1 tablespoon rice wine or dry sherry (optional)

1 teaspoon sugar

1/2 teaspoon crushed red pepper

1 tablespoon canola oil, divided

1 clove garlic, minced

1-1/2 cups fresh pea pods, diagonally sliced

1 cup thinly sliced green or red bell pepper

1 pound boneless skinless chicken breasts, cut into 1/2-inch pieces

1 cup thinly sliced red or green cabbage

2 green onions, thinly sliced

1. Cook noodles in boiling water 4 to 5 minutes or until tender. Drain; set aside.

2. Combine chicken broth, soy sauce, vinegar, rice wine, if desired, sugar and red pepper in small bowl; set aside.

3. Heat 1 teaspoon oil in large nonstick skillet or wok. Add garlic, pea pods and bell pepper; cook 1 to 2 minutes or until vegetables are crisp-tender. Remove from skillet; set aside.

4. Heat remaining 2 teaspoons oil in skillet. Add chicken; cook 3 to 4 minutes or until chicken is no longer pink.

5. Add cabbage, cooked vegetables and noodles to skillet. Stir in sauce; toss until well blended. Cook and stir 1 to 2 minutes or until heated through. Sprinkle with green onions before serving.   *Makes 6 servings*

Nutrients per Serving: 1-1/3 cups Salad

Calories 164	**Fiber** 2g
Fat 6g (sat 1g)	**Cholesterol** 45mg
Protein 17g	**Sodium** 353mg
Carbohydrate 12g	

Exchanges: 1/2 starch, 1 vegetable, 2 lean meat

৯ ৯ ৯

Vegetable Napoleon

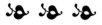

1 teaspoon salt-free garlic and herb seasoning

1/4 teaspoon black pepper

1/4 teaspoon garlic powder

1 large yellow summer squash, thinly sliced lengthwise

1 large zucchini, thinly sliced lengthwise

1/4 cup (1 ounce) shredded reduced-fat mozzarella cheese

1 large tomato, thinly sliced*

For easier slicing, use a serrated bread knife to slice tomatoes.

1. Preheat oven to 350°F. Lightly spray small loaf pan with nonstick cooking spray. Combine seasoning mix, pepper and garlic powder in small bowl.

2. Place one layer of squash and zucchini in bottom of prepared loaf pan. Sprinkle with 1/3 of seasoning mixture and 1 tablespoon cheese. Layer tomato slices over squash. Top with 1/3 of seasoning mixture and 1 tablespoon of cheese. Top with remaining squash, seasoning mixture and cheese. Bake 35 minutes or until vegetables are tender and cheese is melted. Remove from oven and cool slightly before slicing.   *Makes 2 servings*

Nutrients per Serving: 1/2 of total recipe

Calories 78	**Fiber** 3g
Fat 2g (sat 1g)	**Cholesterol** 6mg
Protein 6g	**Sodium** 105mg
Carbohydrate 9g	

Exchanges: 2 vegetable, 1/2 lean meat

Hot Chinese Chicken Salad

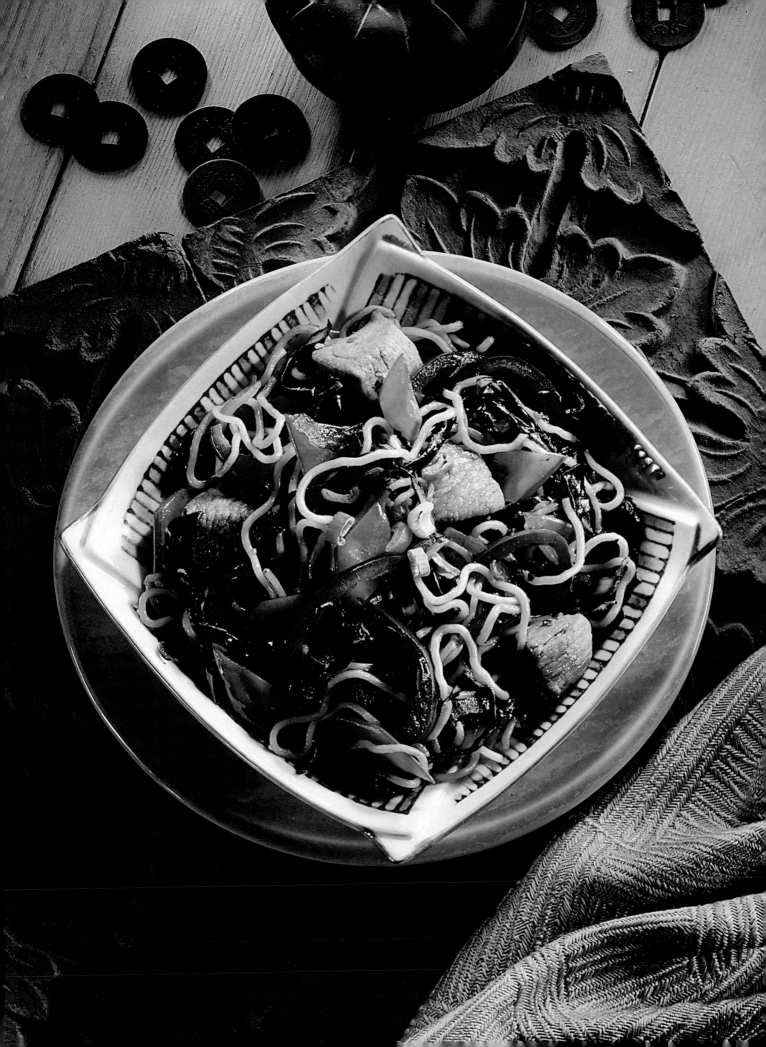

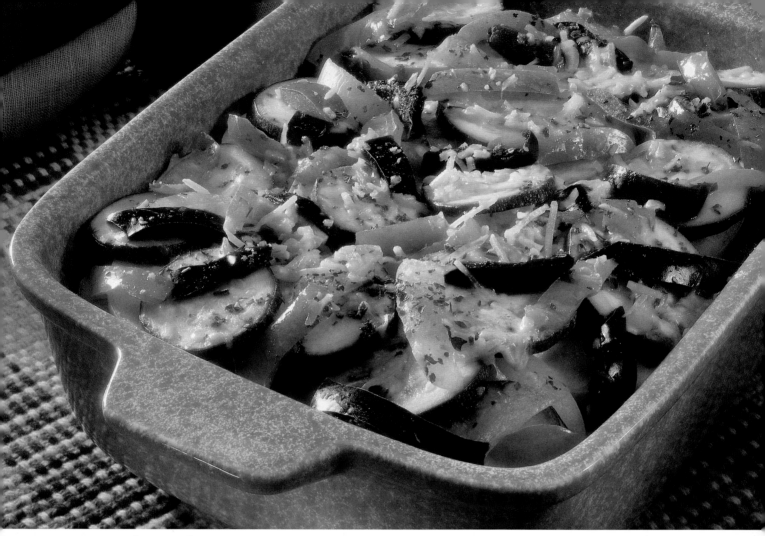

Pepper and Squash Gratin

Pepper and Squash Gratin

low fat · meatless

(Pictured above)

3/4 pound russet potatoes, unpeeled

1/2 pound yellow summer squash, thinly sliced

1/2 pound zucchini, thinly sliced

2 cups frozen pepper stir-fry blend, thawed

1 teaspoon dried oregano leaves

1/2 teaspoon salt
   Black pepper

1/2 cup grated Parmesan cheese or shredded reduced-fat sharp Cheddar cheese

1 tablespoon butter or margarine, cut into 8 pieces

1. Preheat oven to 375°F. Coat 11×7-inch glass baking dish with nonstick cooking spray.

2. Pierce potato several times with fork. Microwave at HIGH 3 minutes; cut into thin slices. Layer half of potatoes, yellow squash, zucchini, pepper stir-fry blend, oregano, salt, black pepper and cheese in prepared baking dish. Repeat layers and top with butter.

3. Cover tightly with foil; bake 25 minutes or until vegetables are just tender. Remove foil and bake 10 minutes or until lightly browned.

Makes 8 servings

Note: This recipe was tested in an 1100-watt microwave oven.

Nutrients per Serving: 3/4 cup Gratin

Calories 106	**Fiber** 2g
Fat 3g (sat 2g)	**Cholesterol** 8mg
Protein 4g	**Sodium** 267mg
Carbohydrate 15g	

Exchanges: 1 starch, 1/2 fat

South-of-the-Border Baked Potato Topper

meatless

Quick Recipe

1-1/2 teaspoons butter or margarine
1 cup broccoli florets
1 clove garlic, minced
1/2 teaspoon ground cumin
1/2 cup (2 ounces) shredded reduced-fat Monterey Jack cheese
1/4 cup reduced-fat mayonnaise
1/4 cup reduced-fat sour cream
1/4 teaspoon salt
1/8 teaspoon black pepper
4 large hot baked potatoes, cut into halves
Chili powder (optional)

1. Melt butter in medium saucepan over medium heat. Add broccoli, garlic and cumin. Cook and stir 3 to 4 minutes or until broccoli is crisp-tender. Remove from heat and cool slightly.

2. Add cheese, mayonnaise and sour cream to saucepan. Stir well to blend. Add salt and pepper to taste.

3. Spoon mixture over hot baked potato halves and sprinkle with chili powder, if desired.

Makes 8 servings

Nutrients per Serving: 1 topped Baked Potato half

Calories 145	**Fiber** 2g
Fat 6g (sat 3g)	**Cholesterol** 11mg
Protein 4g	**Sodium** 187mg
Carbohydrate 19g	

Exchanges: 1 starch, 1 vegetable, 1 fat

Salmon and Green Bean Salad with Pasta

low fat

Quick Recipe

1 can (6 ounces) red salmon
8 ounces uncooked small whole wheat or regular pasta shells
3/4 cup fresh thin green beans, cut into 2-inch pieces
2/3 cup finely chopped carrots
1/2 cup fat-free cottage cheese
3 tablespoons plain fat-free yogurt
1-1/2 tablespoons lemon juice
1 tablespoon chopped fresh dill
2 teaspoons grated onion
1 teaspoon Dijon mustard

1. Drain salmon and separate into chunks; set aside.

2. Cook pasta according to package directions, including 1/4 teaspoon salt; add green beans during last 6 to 7 minutes of cooking. Drain; rinse under cold running water until pasta and green beans are cool. Drain.

3. Combine pasta, green beans, carrots and salmon in medium bowl.

4. Place cottage cheese, yogurt, lemon juice, dill, onion and mustard in food processor or blender; process until smooth. Pour over pasta mixture; toss to coat evenly.

Makes 6 servings

Nutrients per Serving: about 1 cup

Calories 210	**Fiber** 2g
Fat 3g (sat 1g)	**Cholesterol** 15mg
Protein 16g	**Sodium** 223mg
Carbohydrate 29g	

Exchanges: 1-1/2 starch, 1/2 vegetable, 1-1/2 lean meat

Crab Spinach Salad with Tarragon Dressing

Quick Recipe   *(Pictured at right)*

12 ounces coarsely flaked cooked crabmeat *or* **2 packages (6 ounces each) frozen crabmeat, thawed and drained**

1 cup chopped tomatoes

1 cup sliced cucumber

1/3 cup sliced red onion

1/4 cup fat-free salad dressing or mayonnaise

1/4 cup reduced-fat sour cream

1/4 cup chopped fresh parsley

2 tablespoons fat-free milk

2 teaspoons chopped fresh tarragon *or* **1/2 teaspoon dried tarragon leaves**

1 clove garlic, minced

1/4 teaspoon hot pepper sauce

8 cups torn washed stemmed spinach

1. Combine crabmeat, tomatoes, cucumber and onion in medium bowl.

2. Combine salad dressing, sour cream, parsley, milk, tarragon, garlic and hot pepper sauce in small bowl.

3. Line 4 salad plates with spinach. Place crabmeat mixture evenly over spinach; drizzle with dressing.   *Makes 4 servings*

Nutrients per Serving: 1 cup Salad with 1-1/2 tablespoons Dressing and 2 cups Spinach

Calories 170	**Fiber** 4g
Fat 4g (sat <1g)	**Cholesterol** 91mg
Protein 22g	**Sodium** 481mg
Carbohydrate 14g	

Exchanges: 3 vegetable, 2 lean meat

Marinated Vegetables

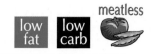

1/4 cup rice wine vinegar or white wine vinegar

3 tablespoons reduced-sodium soy sauce

2 tablespoons fresh lemon juice

1 tablespoon canola oil

1 clove garlic, minced

1 teaspoon minced fresh ginger

1/2 teaspoon sugar

2 cups broccoli florets

2 cups cauliflower florets

2 cups diagonally sliced carrots (1/2-inch pieces)

1/2 pound whole fresh mushrooms

1 large red bell pepper, cut into 1-inch pieces

Lettuce leaves

1. Combine vinegar, soy sauce, lemon juice, oil, garlic, ginger and sugar in large bowl. Set aside.

2. To blanch broccoli, cauliflower and carrots, cook 1 minute in enough salted boiling water to cover. Remove and plunge into cold water, then drain immediately. Toss with oil mixture while still warm. Cool to room temperature.

3. Add mushrooms and bell pepper to bowl; toss to coat. Cover and marinate in refrigerator at least 4 hours or up to 24 hours.

4. Drain vegetables; reserve marinade. Arrange vegetables on lettuce-lined platter. Serve chilled or at room temperature with wooden toothpicks. If desired, serve remaining marinade in small cup for dipping.   *Makes 12 servings*

Nutrients per Serving: about 3/4 cup Vegetables

Calories 37	**Fiber** 2g
Fat 1g (sat <1g)	**Cholesterol** 0mg
Protein 2g	**Sodium** 146mg
Carbohydrate 6g	

Exchanges: 1-1/2 vegetable

Crab Spinach Salad with Tarragon Dressing

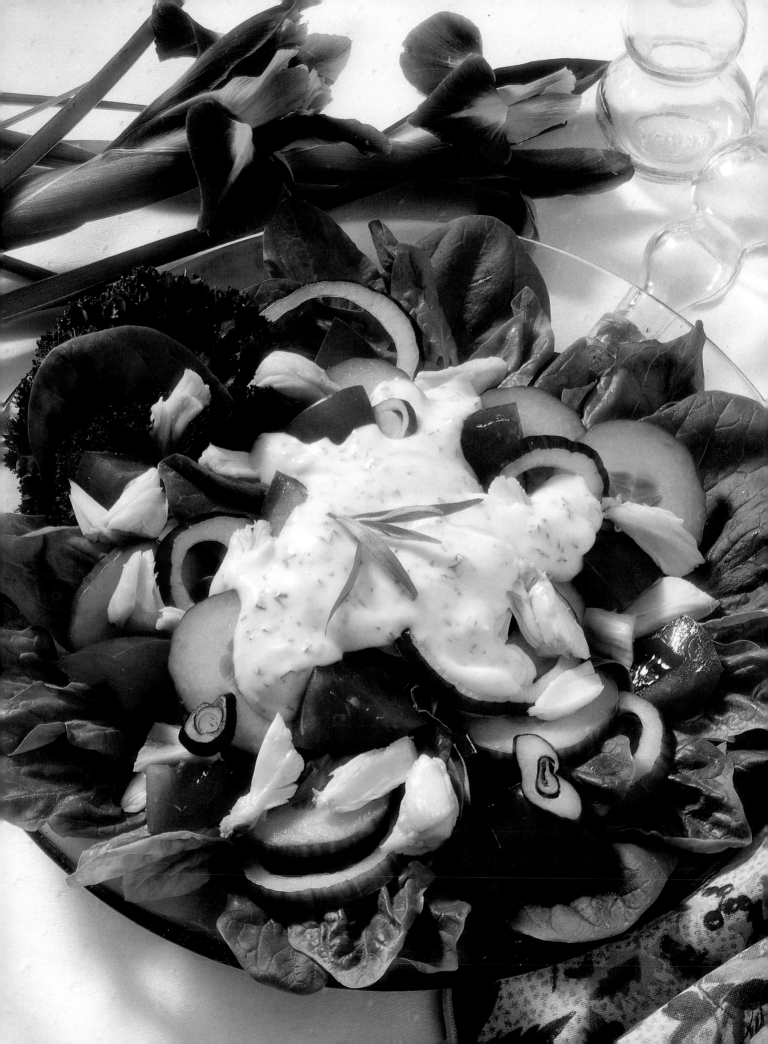

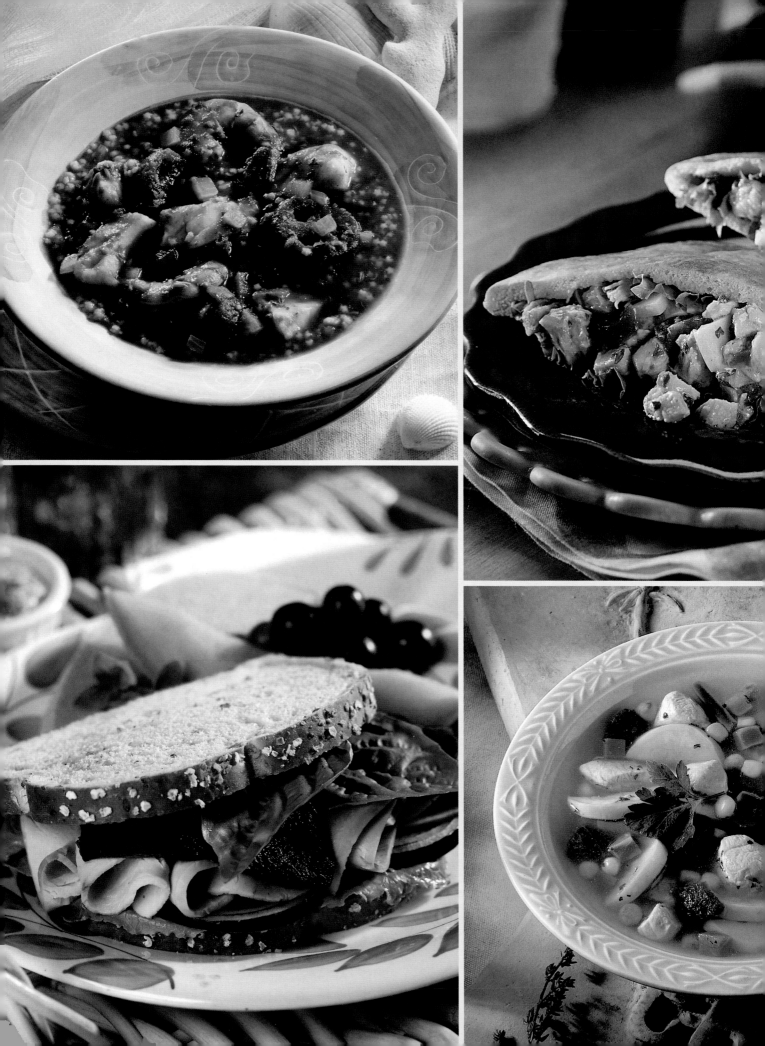

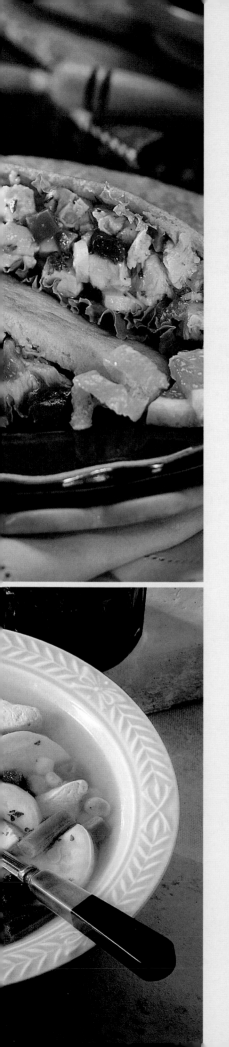

Soups & Sandwiches

❧ ❧ ❧

Tangy Italian Chicken Sandwiches

Quick Recipe   *(Pictured at left)*

> 2 cups (8 ounces) chopped cooked chicken or turkey breast
> 1/3 cup drained bottled hot or mild pickled vegetables (jardinière)
> 2 ounces reduced-fat provolone cheese slices, diced
> 1/4 cup chopped fresh parsley
> 3 tablespoons prepared reduced-fat Italian salad dressing
> 1/4 teaspoon dried oregano leaves
> 4 pita bread rounds (2 ounces each)
> 8 leaves romaine or red leaf lettuce

1. Combine chicken, vegetables, cheese, parsley, dressing and oregano in medium bowl; mix well.

2. Cut each pita in half crosswise; gently open. Line each pocket with lettuce leaf and fill with 1/8 of chicken mixture.

Makes 4 servings

Nutrients per Serving: 2 filled pita halves

Calories 327	**Fiber** 2g
Fat 6g (sat 2g)	**Cholesterol** 58mg
Protein 31g	**Sodium** 840mg
Carbohydrate 35g	

Exchanges: 2 starch, 1 vegetable, 3 lean meat

Clockwise from top left: *Mediterranean Fish Soup (page 148), Tangy Italian Chicken Sandwiches, Bounty Soup (page 133) and Turkey Sandwich with Roasted Bell Peppers (page 140)*

Kansas City Steak Soup

high fiber

Quick Recipe   *(Pictured at right)*

Nonstick cooking spray
1/2 pound 95% lean ground beef
1 cup chopped onion
3 cups frozen mixed vegetables
2 cups water
1 can (14-1/2 ounces) stewed tomatoes, undrained
1 cup sliced celery
1 beef bouillon cube
1/2 to 1 teaspoon black pepper
1 can (10-1/2 ounces) condensed fat-free beef broth, undiluted
1/2 cup all-purpose flour

1. Spray Dutch oven with cooking spray. Heat over medium-high heat until hot. Add beef and onion. Cook and stir 5 minutes or until beef is browned.

2. Add vegetables, water, tomatoes with juice, celery, bouillon cube and pepper. Bring to a boil. Whisk together beef broth and flour until smooth; add to beef mixture, stirring constantly.

3. Return mixture to a boil. Reduce heat to low. Cover and simmer 15 minutes, stirring frequently.   *Makes 6 servings*

Note: If time permits, allow the soup to simmer an additional 30 minutes. The flavors just get better and better!

Nutrients per Serving: 1-2/3 cups Soup

Calories 198	**Fiber** 5g
Fat 5g (sat 2g)	**Cholesterol** 23mg
Protein 13g	**Sodium** 598mg
Carbohydrate 27g	

Exchanges: 1/2 starch, 3-1/2 vegetable, 1 lean meat, 1/2 fat

Southwestern Sloppy Joes

Quick Recipe

1 pound 95% lean ground beef
1 cup chopped onion
1/4 cup chopped celery
1/4 cup water
1 can (10 ounces) diced tomatoes and green chilies, undrained
1 can (8 ounces) no-salt-added tomato sauce
4 teaspoons brown sugar
1/2 teaspoon ground cumin
1/4 teaspoon salt
9 whole wheat hamburger buns

1. Heat large nonstick skillet over high heat. Add beef, onion, celery and water. Reduce heat to medium. Cook and stir 5 minutes or until meat is no longer pink. Drain fat.

2. Stir in tomatoes and green chilies with juice, tomato sauce, brown sugar, cumin and salt; bring to a boil over high heat. Reduce heat; simmer 20 minutes or until mixture thickens. Serve on whole wheat buns. Garnish as desired.   *Makes 9 servings*

Nutrients per Serving: 1 Sloppy Joe sandwich (1 bun with 1/3 cup meat mixture)

Calories 190	**Fiber** 1g
Fat 4g (sat 1g)	**Cholesterol** 15mg
Protein 13g	**Sodium** 413mg
Carbohydrate 26g	

Exchanges: 1-1/2 starch, 1 vegetable, 1 lean meat

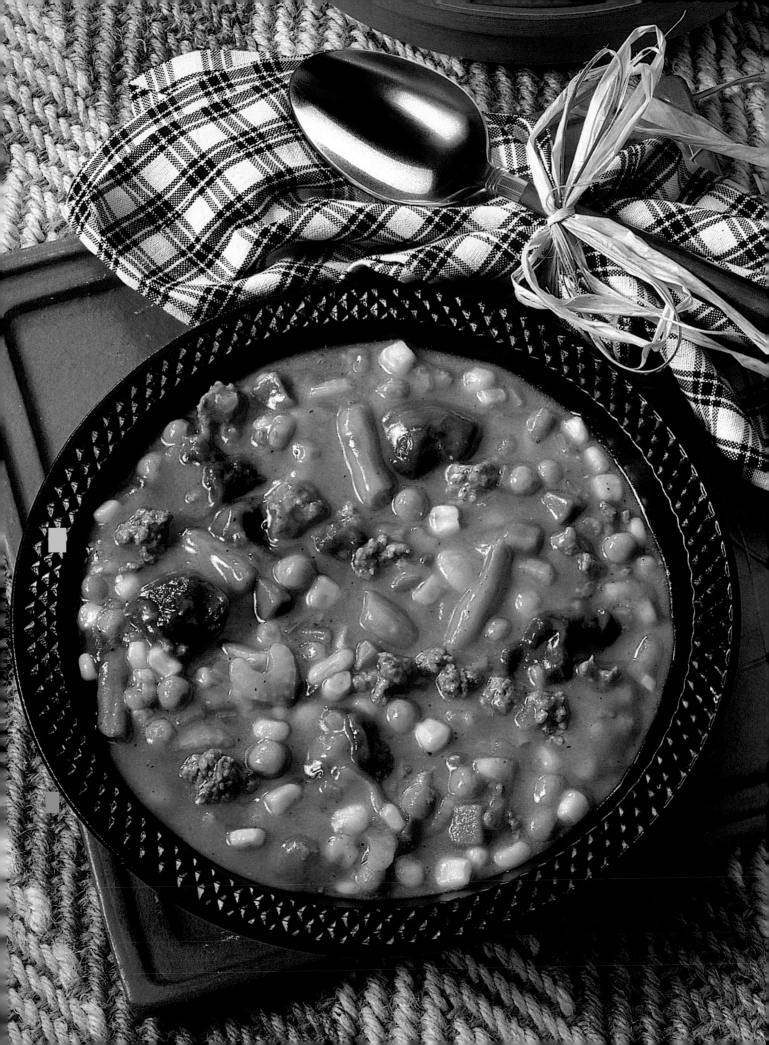

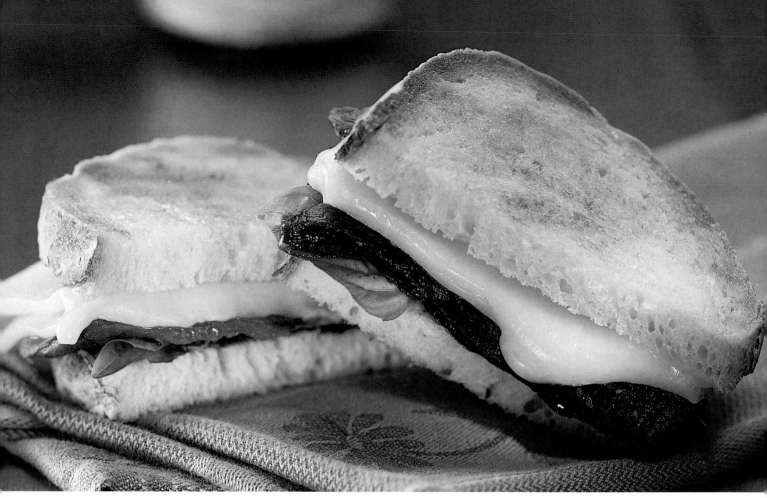

Grilled Mozzarella & Roasted Red Pepper Sandwich

Grilled Mozzarella & Roasted Red Pepper Sandwich

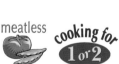

meatless

cooking for 1 or 2

Quick Recipe   *(Pictured above)*

1 tablespoon reduced-fat olive oil vinaigrette or prepared reduced-fat Italian salad dressing

2 slices (1 ounce each) Italian-style sandwich bread

1/3 cup bottled roasted sweet red peppers, rinsed, drained and patted dry

Fresh basil leaves (optional)

2 slices (1 ounce each) part-skim mozzarella or reduced-fat Swiss cheese

Olive oil-flavored nonstick cooking spray

1. Brush dressing on one side of one slice of bread; top with peppers, basil, if desired, cheese and second bread slice. Lightly spray both sides of sandwich with cooking spray.

2. Heat skillet over medium heat until hot. Place sandwich in skillet and grill 4 to 5 minutes on each side or until brown and cheese is melted. Cut in half before serving, if desired.   *Makes 1 serving*

Nutrients per Serving: 1 Sandwich (2 Sandwich halves)

Calories 303	**Fiber** 2g
Fat 9g (sat 5g)	**Cholesterol** 25mg
Protein 16g	**Sodium** 727mg
Carbohydrate 35g	

Exchanges: 2 starch, 1 vegetable, 1 lean meat, 1-1/2 fat

Bounty Soup

high
fiber

Quick Recipe   *(Pictured on page 128)*

- 1 to 2 yellow crookneck squash
  (1/2 pound), cut in half lengthwise,
  then crosswise into 1/4-inch slices
- 2 cups frozen mixed vegetables
- 1 teaspoon dried parsley flakes
- 1/8 teaspoon salt
- 1/8 teaspoon dried rosemary leaves
- 1/8 teaspoon dried thyme leaves
- 1/8 teaspoon black pepper
- 2 teaspoons vegetable oil
- 3 boneless skinless chicken breasts (about
  3/4 pound), chopped
- 1 can (14-1/2 ounces) fat-free reduced-
  sodium chicken broth
- 1 can (14-1/2 ounces) stewed tomatoes,
  undrained

1. Place squash, mixed vegetables, parsley, salt, rosemary, thyme and pepper in medium bowl.

2. Heat oil in large saucepan over medium-high heat. Add chicken; stir-fry 2 minutes. Stir in vegetables with seasonings. Add broth and tomatoes with juice, breaking large tomatoes apart. Cover; bring to a boil. Reduce heat to low. Cover; cook 5 minutes or until vegetables are tender.   *Makes 4 servings*

Nutrients per Serving: 1-1/2 cups Soup

Calories 225	**Fiber** 6g
Fat 4g (sat 1g)	**Cholesterol** 60mg
Protein 27g	**Sodium** 490mg
Carbohydrate 20g	

Exchanges: 4 vegetable, 2-1/2 lean meat

Chicken and Grape Pita Sandwiches

Quick Recipe

- 1/2 cup plain fat-free yogurt
- 1/4 cup reduced-fat mayonnaise
- 2 tablespoons fresh tarragon leaves,
  minced, *or* 2 teaspoons dried
  tarragon leaves
- 2 teaspoons Dijon mustard
- 2 teaspoons honey
- 1/2 teaspoon black pepper
- 3 cups cubed cooked chicken breast
- 1 cup thinly sliced celery
- 1 cup red seedless grapes, cut into halves
- 1 medium head red leaf lettuce, washed
- 3 pita bread rounds (2 ounces each)

1. Combine yogurt, mayonnaise, tarragon, mustard, honey and pepper in large bowl until blended. Add chicken, celery and grapes; stir to coat with dressing.

2. Separate lettuce leaves. Select 6 large leaves and discard stems. Tear or shred remaining leaves.

3. Cut each pita in half crosswise; gently open. Line each pocket with 1 large lettuce leaf. Add handful of torn leaves to each pita. Spoon about 2/3 cup chicken mixture into each pita.

Makes 6 servings

Nutrients per Serving: 1 Sandwich (1/2 Pita round with lettuce and 2/3 cup Chicken mixture)

Calories 249	**Fiber** 1g
Fat 6g (sat 1g)	**Cholesterol** 50mg
Protein 22g	**Sodium** 278mg
Carbohydrate 28g	

Exchanges: 1 starch, 1/2 fruit, 1 vegetable,
2-1/2 lean meat

Asian Wraps

Quick Recipe (Pictured at right)

high fiber

Nonstick cooking spray

8 ounces boneless skinless chicken breasts or thighs, cut into 1/2-inch pieces

1 teaspoon minced fresh ginger

1 teaspoon minced fresh garlic

1/4 teaspoon red pepper flakes

1/4 cup reduced-sodium teriyaki sauce

4 cups packaged coleslaw mix (about 8 ounces)

1/2 cup sliced green onions

4 flour tortillas (10 inches)

8 teaspoons no-sugar-added plum fruit spread

1. Spray nonstick wok or large nonstick skillet with cooking spray; heat over medium-high heat. Stir-fry chicken 2 minutes.

2. Add ginger, garlic and red pepper flakes; stir-fry 2 minutes.

3. Add teriyaki sauce; mix well.* Add coleslaw mix and green onions; stir-fry 4 minutes or until chicken is no longer pink and cabbage is crisp-tender.

4. Spread each tortilla with 2 teaspoons fruit spread. Evenly spoon chicken mixture down center of tortillas. Roll up to form wraps.

Makes 4 servings

If sauce is too thick, add up to 2 tablespoons water to thin it.

Nutrients per Serving: 1 Wrap

Calories 367	**Fiber** 5g
Fat 6g (sat 1g)	**Cholesterol** 33mg
Protein 22g	**Sodium** 830mg
Carbohydrate 57g	

Exchanges: 3 starch, 2 vegetable, 2 lean meat

Chunky Chicken Stew

high fiber cooking for 1 or 2

Quick Recipe

1 teaspoon olive oil

1 small onion, chopped

1 cup thinly sliced carrots

1 cup fat-free reduced-sodium chicken broth

1 can (14-1/2 ounces) no-salt-added diced tomatoes, undrained

1 cup diced cooked chicken breast

3 cups sliced kale or baby spinach leaves

1. Heat oil in large saucepan over medium-high heat. Add onion; cook and stir about 5 minutes or until golden brown, stirring occasionally.

2. Stir in carrots, then broth; bring to a boil. Reduce heat and simmer, uncovered, 5 minutes.

3. Add tomatoes; simmer 5 minutes or until carrots are tender. Add chicken; heat through.

4. Add kale, stirring until kale is wilted. Simmer 1 minute. Ladle evenly into 2 soup bowls.

Makes 2 servings

Nutrients per Serving: 1 bowl Stew (1/2 of total recipe)

Calories 274	**Fiber** 7g
Fat 6g (sat 1g)	**Cholesterol** 0mg
Protein 30g	**Sodium** 209mg
Carbohydrate 25g	

Exchanges: 5 vegetable, 3 lean meat

Asian Wraps

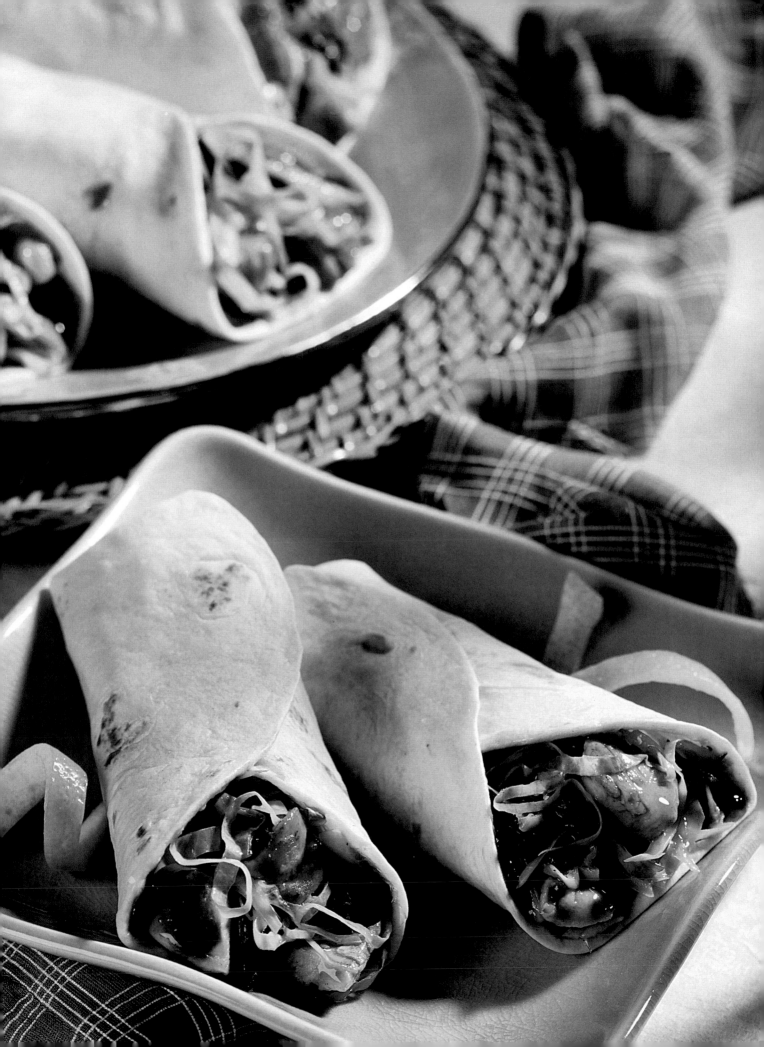

Cioppino

(Pictured at right)

- 1 teaspoon olive oil
- 1 large onion, chopped
- 1 cup sliced celery, with celery tops
- 1 clove garlic, minced
- 4 cups water
- 1 fish, chicken or vegetable bouillon cube
- 1 tablespoon salt-free Italian herb seasoning
- 1/4 pound cod or other boneless mild-flavored fish fillets
- 1 large tomato, chopped
- 1/4 pound uncooked small shrimp, peeled and deveined
- 1/4 pound uncooked bay scallops
- 1/4 cup flaked crabmeat or crabmeat blend
- 1 can (10 ounces) baby clams, rinsed and drained (optional)
- 2 tablespoons fresh lemon juice
- Lemon wedges (optional)

1. Heat olive oil in large saucepan over medium heat until hot. Add onion, celery and garlic. Cook and stir 5 minutes or until onion is soft. Add water, bouillon cube and Italian seasoning. Cover and bring to a boil over high heat.

2. Cut cod fillets into 1/2-inch pieces. Add cod and tomato to saucepan. Reduce heat to medium-low; simmer 10 to 15 minutes or until seafood is opaque. Add shrimp, scallops, crabmeat, clams, if desired, and lemon juice. Heat through. Shrimp should be opaque. Garnish with lemon wedges, if desired.

Makes 4 servings

Nutrients per Serving: 1-3/4 cups Cioppino

Calories 122	**Fiber** 2g
Fat 2g (sat <1g)	**Cholesterol** 75mg
Protein 18g	**Sodium** 412mg
Carbohydrate 8g	

Exchanges: 1 vegetable, 2 lean meat

Huevos Ranchwich

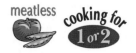

Quick Recipe

- 1/4 cup EGG BEATERS® Healthy Real Egg Product
- 1 teaspoon diced green chiles
- 1 whole wheat hamburger roll, split and toasted
- 1 tablespoon thick and chunky salsa, heated
- 1 tablespoon shredded reduced-fat Cheddar and Monterey Jack cheese blend

On lightly greased griddle or skillet, pour Egg Beaters® into lightly greased 4-inch egg ring or biscuit cutter. Sprinkle with chiles. Cook 2 to 3 minutes or until bottom of egg patty is set. Remove egg ring and turn egg patty over. Cook 1 to 2 minutes longer or until done.

To serve, place egg patty on bottom of roll. Top with salsa, cheese and roll top.

Makes 1 sandwich

Nutrients per Serving: 1 sandwich

Calories 168	**Fiber** 2g
Fat 4g (sat 1g)	**Cholesterol** 5mg
Protein 13g	**Sodium** 495mg
Carbohydrate 21g	

Exchanges: 1-1/2 starch, 1 lean meat

Cioppino

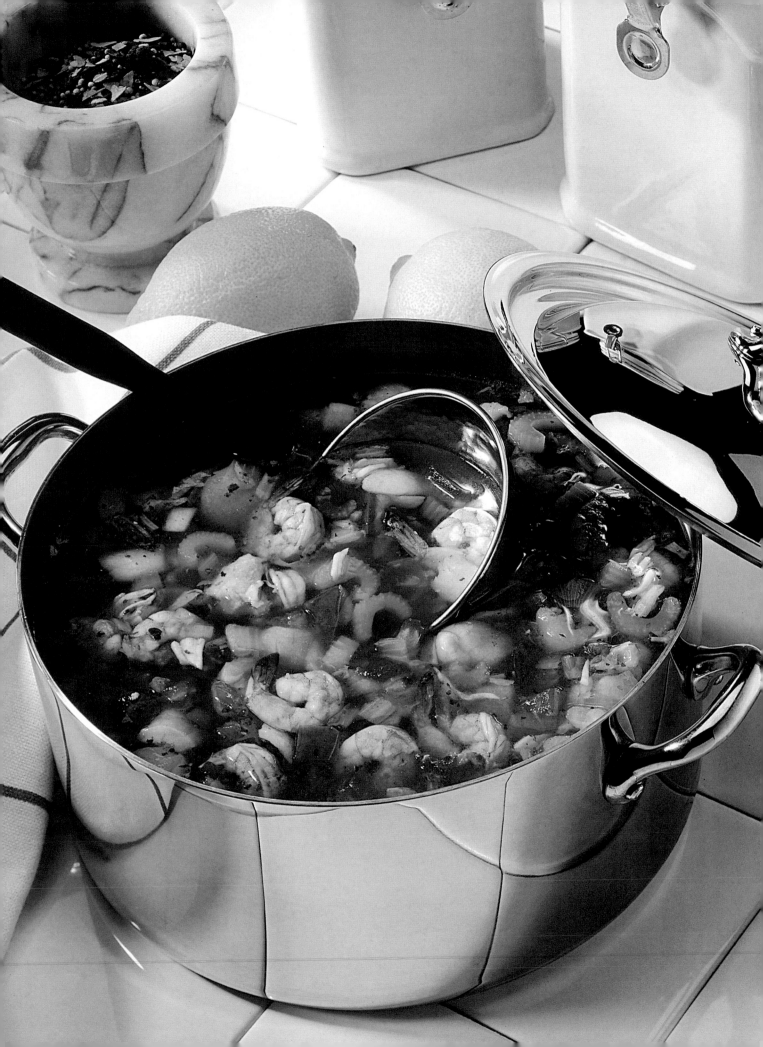

Grilled Flank Steak with Horseradish Sauce

(Pictured at right)

- 1 pound beef flank steak
- 2 tablespoons reduced-sodium soy sauce
- 1 tablespoon red wine vinegar or cider vinegar
- 2 cloves garlic, minced
- 1/2 teaspoon black pepper
- 1 cup fat-free sour cream
- 1 tablespoon prepared horseradish
- 1 tablespoon Dijon mustard
- 1/4 cup finely chopped fresh parsley
- 1/2 teaspoon salt
- 6 sourdough rolls (2 ounces each), split
- 6 romaine lettuce leaves
- Small pickles (optional)

1. Place flank steak in large resealable plastic food storage bag. Add soy sauce, vinegar, garlic and pepper. Close bag securely; turn to coat. Marinate in refrigerator at least 1 hour.

2. Prepare grill or preheat broiler. Drain steak; discard marinade. Grill or broil steak over medium-high heat 5 minutes. Turn beef; grill 6 minutes for medium-rare or until desired doneness. Remove from grill. Cover with foil; let stand 10 minutes. Thinly slice steak across grain.

3. Combine sour cream, horseradish, mustard, parsley and salt in small bowl until well blended. Spread rolls with horseradish sauce; layer with sliced steak and lettuce. Garnish with small pickles, if desired.   *Makes 6 servings*

Nutrients per Serving: 1 sandwich (1 roll with 2 ounces cooked beef, 3 tablespoons plus 1 teaspoon Horseradish Sauce and 1 lettuce leaf)

Calories 307	**Fiber** 1g
Fat 9g (sat 3g)	**Cholesterol** 32mg
Protein 24g	**Sodium** 600mg
Carbohydrate 29g	

Exchanges: 2 starch, 3 lean meat

Quick Quesadillas

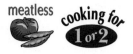

Quick Recipe

- 1 flour tortilla (6 inch)
- 1 KRAFT® 2% Milk Singles Process Cheese Food with Added Calcium
- 1 tablespoon chopped red pepper
- 1 teaspoon sliced green onion

TOP tortilla with 2% Milk Singles and vegetables. Fold in half. Place on microwavable plate.

MICROWAVE on HIGH 15 to 20 seconds or until 2% Milk Singles begin to melt. Fold in half again.   *Makes 1 serving*

Nutrients per Serving: 1 Quesadilla

Calories 150	**Fiber** 1g
Fat 5g (sat 3g)	**Cholesterol** 10mg
Protein 7g	**Sodium** 430mg
Carbohydrate 19g	

Exchanges: 1 starch, 1 lean meat

Tip

Horseradish is a large, white root with a pungent flavor. It can sometimes be found fresh in produce markets, but it is most commonly found grated, preserved in vinegar and packed in jars in the refrigerated section of the supermarket. It is referred to as "prepared horseradish" in recipes. Once opened, it loses its pungency quickly, so plan to use it within a few weeks.

Grilled Flank Steak with Horseradish Sauce

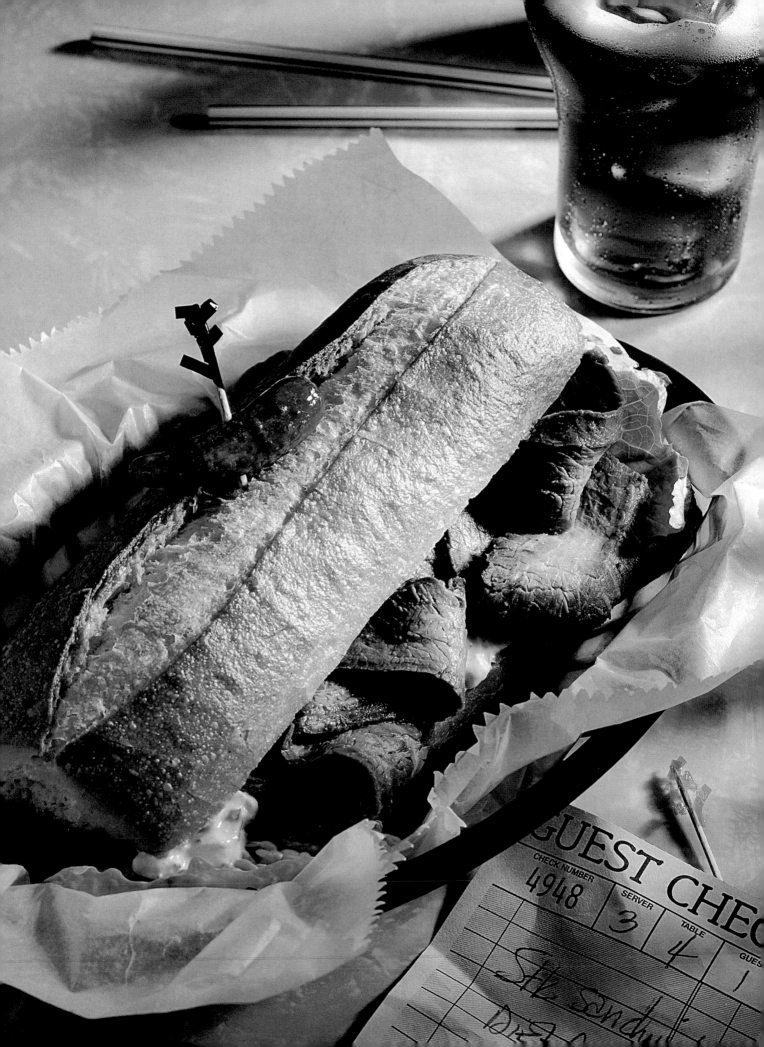

GUEST CHEC

CHECK NUMBER	SERVER	TABLE	GUES
4948	3	4	1

Turkey Sandwiches with Roasted Bell Peppers

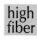

high fiber

Quick Recipe   *(Pictured on page 128)*

> 2 large red bell peppers
> 8 slices whole-grain or millet bread
> 1/4 cup reduced-fat mayonnaise
> 4 romaine lettuce leaves *or* 8 spinach
>   leaves
> 8 ounces thinly sliced skinless roast
>   turkey breast
> 4 thin slices red onion
> 8 large basil leaves (optional)

1. Preheat broiler. Cut bell peppers into quarters; discard stems and seeds. Place peppers, skin sides up, on foil-lined baking sheet. Broil 3 inches from heat 10 minutes or until skin is blackened. Wrap peppers in foil from baking sheet; let stand 10 minutes. Peel off and discard skin.

2. Spread 4 bread slices with mayonnaise. Top evenly with lettuce, turkey, onion and basil, if desired. Arrange peppers over basil; top with remaining bread slices.   *Makes 4 servings*

Nutrients per Serving: 1 Sandwich

Calories 282	**Fiber** 7g
Fat 7g (sat 1g)	**Cholesterol** 47mg
Protein 27g	**Sodium** 282mg
Carbohydrate 37g	

Exchanges: 2-1/2 starch, 2-1/2 lean meat

Tuscan Chicken with White Beans

high fiber

> 1 large fresh fennel bulb (about
>   3/4 pound)
> 1 teaspoon olive oil
> 8 ounces boneless skinless chicken thighs,
>   cut into 3/4-inch pieces
> 1 teaspoon dried rosemary leaves,
>   crushed
> 1/2 teaspoon black pepper
> 1 can (14-1/2 ounces) no-salt-added
>   stewed tomatoes, undrained
> 1 can (14-1/2 ounces) fat-free reduced-
>   sodium chicken broth
> 1 can (16 ounces) cannellini beans, rinsed
>   and drained
> Hot pepper sauce (optional)

1. Cut off and reserve 1/4 cup chopped feathery fennel tops. Chop bulb into 1/2-inch pieces. Heat oil in large saucepan over medium heat. Add chopped fennel bulb; cook 5 minutes, stirring occasionally.

2. Sprinkle chicken with rosemary and pepper. Add to saucepan; cook and stir 2 minutes. Add tomatoes and chicken broth; bring to a boil. Cover and simmer 10 minutes.

3. Stir in beans; simmer, uncovered, 15 minutes or until chicken is cooked through and sauce thickens. Season to taste with hot sauce, if desired. Ladle into 4 shallow bowls; top with reserved fennel tops.   *Makes 4 servings*

Nutrients per Serving: 1-1/2 cups soup

Calories 220	**Fiber** 7g
Fat 7g (sat 2g)	**Cholesterol** 34mg
Protein 16g	**Sodium** 321mg
Carbohydrate 24g	

Exchanges: 1-1/2 starch, 2 lean meat

Turkey Chili with Black Beans

(Pictured below)

- **1 pound ground turkey breast**
- **1 can (14-1/2 ounces) fat-free reduced-sodium chicken broth**
- **1 large onion, finely chopped**
- **1 medium green bell pepper, cored, seeded and diced**
- **2 teaspoons chili powder**
- **1/2 teaspoon ground allspice**
- **1/4 teaspoon ground cinnamon**
- **1/4 teaspoon paprika**
- **1 can (15 ounces) black beans, rinsed**
- **1 can (14-1/2 ounces) crushed tomatoes in tomato purée**
- **2 teaspoons apple cider vinegar**

1. Heat large nonstick skillet over high heat. Add turkey, chicken broth, onion and bell pepper. Cook and stir, breaking up turkey. Cook until turkey is no longer pink.

2. Add chili powder, allspice, cinnamon and paprika. Reduce heat to medium-low; simmer 10 minutes. Add black beans, tomatoes and vinegar; bring to a boil.

3. Reduce heat to low; simmer 20 to 25 minutes or until thickened to desired consistency. Garnish as desired. *Makes 4 servings*

Nutrients per Serving: about 1-1/3 cups Chili

Calories 272	**Fiber** 10g
Fat 2g (sat 0g)	**Cholesterol** 75mg
Protein 40g	**Sodium** 873mg
Carbohydrate 31g	

Exchanges: 1 starch, 3 vegetable, 4 lean meat

Turkey Chili with Black Beans

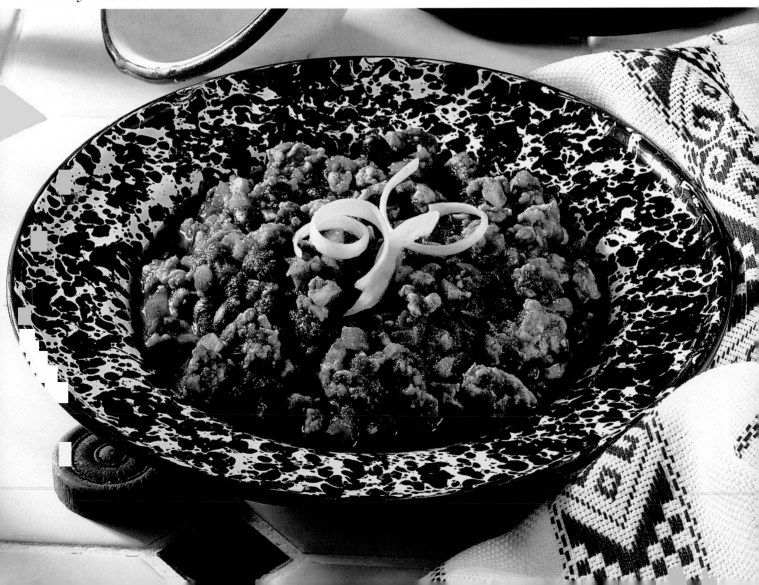

Sassy Southwestern Veggie Wraps

high fiber · meatless · cooking for 1 or 2

Quick Recipe   *(Pictured at right)*

- **1/2 cup diced zucchini**
- **1/2 cup diced red or yellow bell pepper**
- **1/2 cup frozen corn, thawed**
- **1 jalapeño pepper,* seeded and chopped**
- **3/4 cup shredded reduced-fat Mexican cheese blend**
- **3 tablespoons prepared salsa or picante sauce**
- **2 fat-free flour tortillas (8 inches)**

Jalapeño peppers can sting and irritate the skin; wear rubber gloves when handling peppers and do not touch eyes. Wash hands after handling peppers.

1. Combine zucchini, bell pepper, corn and jalapeño pepper in small bowl. Stir in cheese and salsa; mix well.

2. Soften tortillas according to package directions. Spoon vegetable mixture down center of tortillas, distributing evenly; roll up burrito-style. Serve wraps cold or warm.*

Makes 2 servings

*To warm each wrap, cover loosely with plastic wrap and microwave at HIGH 40 to 45 seconds or until cheese is melted.

Nutrients per Serving: 1 Wrap

Calories 221	**Fiber** 8g
Fat 7g (sat 5g)	**Cholesterol** 19mg
Protein 16g	**Sodium** 664mg
Carbohydrate 26g	

Exchanges: 1-1/2 starch, 1 vegetable, 1 lean meat, 1/2 fat

Barbecued Pork Sandwiches

- **2 pork tenderloins (about 1-1/2 pounds total)**
- **1/3 cup prepared barbecue sauce**
- **1/2 cup prepared horseradish**
- **4 pita bread rounds (2 ounces each)**
- **1 medium onion, thinly sliced**
- **4 romaine lettuce leaves**
- **1 medium red bell pepper, cut lengthwise into 1/4-inch-thick slices**
- **1 medium green bell pepper, cut lengthwise into 1/4-inch-thick slices**

1. Preheat oven to 400°F.

2. Place pork tenderloins in roasting pan; brush with barbecue sauce. Bake tenderloins 15 minutes; turn and bake 15 minutes more or until internal temperature reaches 160°F when tested with meat thermometer inserted into thickest part of roast.

3. Transfer roast to cutting board; cover with foil. Let stand 10 minutes before carving.

4. Slice pork across grain. Cut each pita in half crosswise; gently open. Spread horseradish onto insides of halves; stuff evenly with pork, onion, lettuce and bell peppers. Garnish, if desired.

Makes 8 servings

Nutrients per Serving: 1 Sandwich (1 filled pita half) with about 3 ounces Barbecued Pork

Calories 220	**Fiber** 1g
Fat 5g (sat 1g)	**Cholesterol** 61mg
Protein 23g	**Sodium** 314mg
Carbohydrate 23g	

Exchanges: 1 starch, 1 vegetable, 2-1/2 lean meat

Sassy Southwestern Veggie Wrap

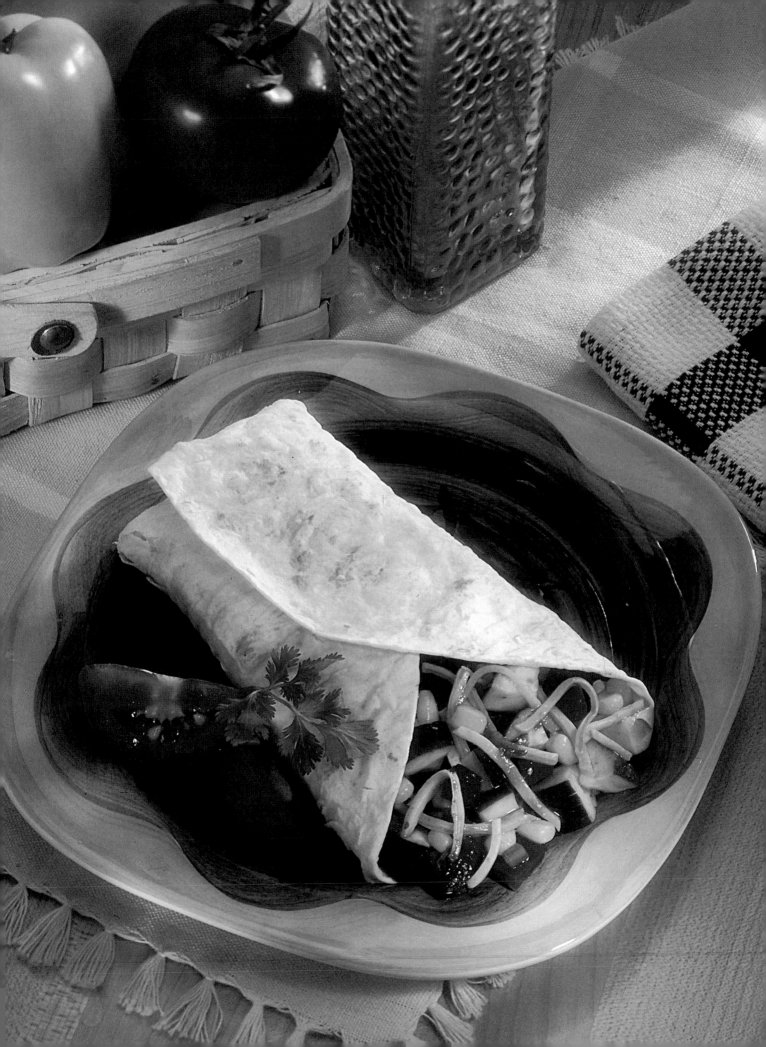

Texas-Style Chili

(Pictured at right)

Nonstick cooking spray
1 pound lean boneless beef chuck, cut into 1/2-inch pieces
2 cups chopped onions
5 cloves garlic, minced
2 tablespoons chili powder
1 tablespoon ground cumin
1 teaspoon ground coriander
1 teaspoon dried oregano leaves
2-1/2 cups fat-free reduced-sodium beef broth
1 cup prepared mild salsa or picante sauce
2 cans (15 ounces each) pinto or red beans (or one of each), rinsed and drained
1/2 cup chopped fresh cilantro
1/2 cup fat-free sour cream
1 cup chopped ripe tomatoes

1. Spray Dutch oven or large saucepan with cooking spray; heat over medium-high heat until hot. Add beef, onions and garlic; cook and stir until beef is no longer pink, about 5 minutes.

2. Sprinkle mixture with chili powder, cumin, coriander and oregano; mix well. Add beef broth and salsa; bring to a boil. Cover; simmer 45 minutes.

3. Stir in beans; continue to simmer, uncovered, 30 minutes or until beef is tender and chili has thickened, stirring occasionally.

4. Stir in cilantro. Ladle into 8 bowls; top evenly with sour cream and tomatoes. Garnish with pickled jalapeño peppers, if desired.

Makes 8 servings

Nutrients per Serving: about 3/4 cup Chili with 1 tablespoon sour cream and 2 tablespoons chopped tomatoes

Calories 268	**Fiber** 2g
Fat 7g (sat 2g)	**Cholesterol** 37mg
Protein 25g	**Sodium** 725mg
Carbohydrate 31g	

Exchanges: 1-1/2 starch, 1-1/2 vegetable, 2-1/2 lean meat

Meatball Grinders

1 pound ground chicken breast
1/2 cup fresh whole wheat or white bread crumbs (1 slice bread)
1 egg white
3 tablespoons finely chopped fresh parsley
2 cloves garlic, minced
1/4 teaspoon salt
1/8 teaspoon black pepper
Nonstick cooking spray
1/4 cup chopped onion
1 can (8 ounces) whole tomatoes, drained and coarsely chopped
1 can (4 ounces) no-salt-added tomato sauce
1 teaspoon dried Italian seasoning
4 small hard rolls, split
2 tablespoons shredded Parmesan cheese

1. Combine chicken, bread crumbs, egg white, parsley, garlic, salt and pepper in medium bowl. Form mixture into 12 to 16 meatballs.

2. Spray medium nonstick skillet with cooking spray; heat over medium heat until hot. Add meatballs; cook and stir about 5 minutes or until browned on all sides. Remove meatballs from skillet.

3. Add onion to skillet; cook and stir 2 to 3 minutes. Stir in tomatoes, tomato sauce and Italian seasoning; heat to a boil. Reduce heat to low and simmer, covered, 15 minutes. Return meatballs to skillet; simmer, covered, 15 minutes.

4. Place 3 to 4 meatballs in each roll. Divide sauce evenly; spoon over meatballs. Sprinkle evenly with cheese. *Makes 4 servings*

Nutrients per Serving: 1 Grinder sandwich

Calories 340	**Fiber** 3g
Fat 7g (sat 2g)	**Cholesterol** 63mg
Protein 31g	**Sodium** 702mg
Carbohydrate 40g	

Exchanges: 2 starch, 1-1/2 vegetable, 3 lean meat

Texas-Style Chili

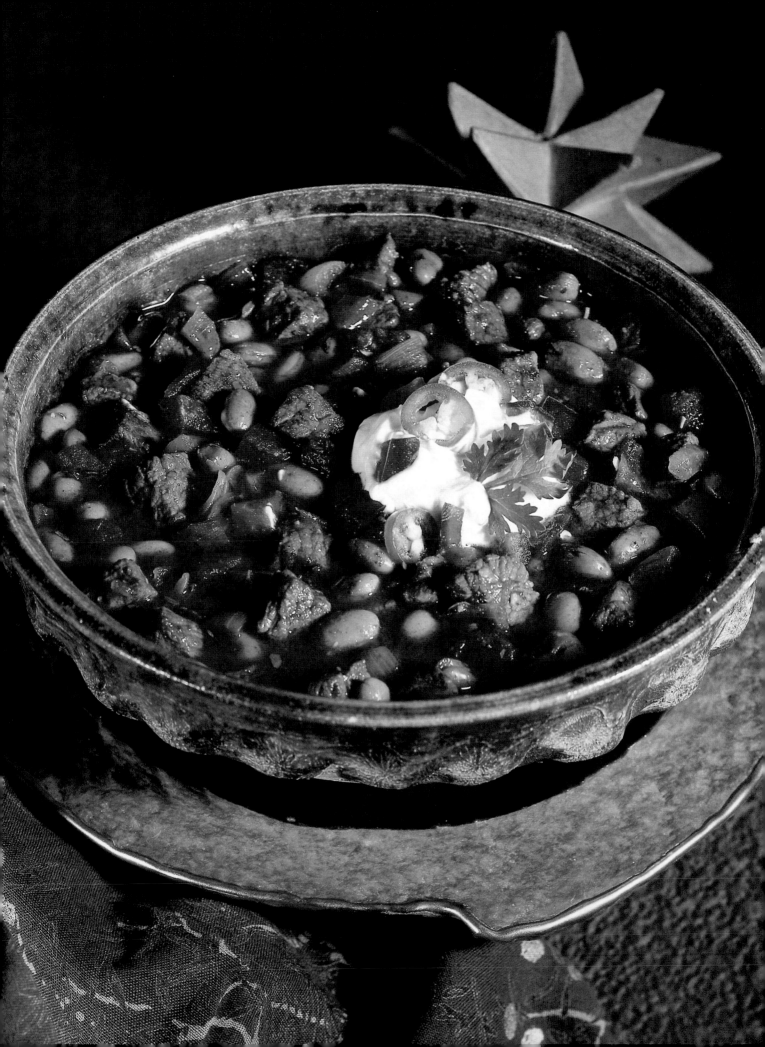

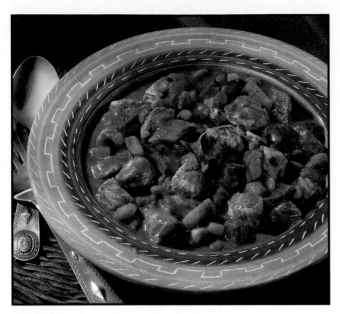

Southwest Turkey Tenderloin Stew

2. Add all remaining ingredients except cilantro; mix well. Cover and cook on LOW 5 hours or until turkey is no longer pink in center and vegetables are crisp-tender. To serve, ladle into 6 bowls. Garnish with cilantro, if desired.

Makes 6 servings

Nutrients per Serving: 1-1/4 cups Stew

Calories 203	**Fiber** 6g
Fat 3g (sat 1g)	**Cholesterol** 45mg
Protein 25g	**Sodium** 827mg
Carbohydrate 23g	

Exchanges: 1 starch, 1-1/2 vegetable, 2-1/2 lean meat

Garden Tuna Salad

Quick Recipe

1 can (6 ounces) tuna packed in water, drained

1 medium carrot, chopped

1 rib celery, chopped

1/2 cup reduced-fat Monterey Jack cheese cubes (1/4 inch)

1/4 cup frozen green peas, thawed and drained

1/4 teaspoon dried parsley flakes

1/3 cup prepared reduced-fat Italian salad dressing

2 pita bread rounds (2 ounces each)

4 lettuce leaves

4 tomato slices

1. Place tuna in large bowl; break into chunks. Add carrot, celery, cheese, peas and parsley; toss to blend. Pour dressing over tuna mixture; toss lightly to coat.

2. Cut each pita in half crosswise; gently open. Place lettuce leaf and tomato slice inside each pocket. Divide tuna salad evenly among pockets.

Makes 4 servings

Nutrients per Serving: 1 pita half with about 1/2 cup Tuna Salad, 1 lettuce leaf and 1 tomato slice

Calories 213	**Fiber** 4g
Fat 6g (sat 2g)	**Cholesterol** 24mg
Protein 19g	**Sodium** 605mg
Carbohydrate 22g	

Exchanges: 1-1/2 starch, 2 lean meat

Southwest Turkey Tenderloin Stew

(Pictured above)

1 package (about 1-1/2 pounds) turkey tenderloins, cut into 3/4-inch pieces

1 tablespoon chili powder

1 teaspoon ground cumin

1/4 teaspoon salt

1 medium red bell pepper, cut into 3/4-inch pieces

1 medium green bell pepper, cut into 3/4-inch pieces

3/4 cup chopped red or yellow onion

3 cloves garlic, minced

1 can (15-1/2 ounces) chili beans in spicy sauce, undrained

1 can (14-1/2 ounces) chili-style stewed tomatoes, undrained

3/4 cup prepared mild salsa or picante sauce

Fresh cilantro (optional)

Slow Cooker Directions

1. Place turkey in slow cooker. Sprinkle chili powder, cumin and salt over turkey; toss to coat.

Jamaican Chicken Sandwich

- 1 teaspoon Jerk Seasoning (recipe follows)
- 4 boneless skinless chicken breasts (about 1 pound)
- 2 tablespoons reduced-fat mayonnaise
- 2 tablespoons plain fat-free yogurt
- 1 tablespoon mango chutney
- 4 onion rolls (2 ounces each), split and toasted
- 4 lettuce leaves
- 8 slices peeled mango or papaya

1. Prepare Jerk Seasoning. Sprinkle chicken with jerk seasoning and set aside. Spray grid with nonstick cooking spray. Prepare grill for direct cooking.

2. Place chicken on grid, 3 to 4 inches from medium-hot coals. Grill 5 to 7 minutes on each side or until no longer pink in center.

3. Combine mayonnaise, yogurt and chutney in small bowl; spread onto onion rolls.

4. Place chicken on onion roll bottoms; top each with lettuce leaf and 2 slices of fruit.

Makes 4 servings

Jerk Seasoning

- 1-1/2 teaspoons salt
- 1-1/2 teaspoons ground allspice
- 1 teaspoon sugar
- 1 teaspoon ground thyme leaves
- 1 teaspoon black pepper
- 1/2 teaspoon garlic powder
- 1/2 teaspoon ground red pepper
- 1/4 teaspoon ground cinnamon
- 1/4 teaspoon ground nutmeg

Combine all ingredients in small bowl.

Nutrients per Serving: 1 Sandwich (1 roll with 1 Chicken breast, 1 tablespoon chutney spread, 1 lettuce leaf and 2 mango slices)

Calories 302	**Fiber** 1g	
Fat 8g (sat 2g)	**Cholesterol** 72mg	
Protein 30g	**Sodium** 373mg	
Carbohydrate 28g		

Exchanges: 1-1/2 starch, 1/2 fruit, 3 lean meat

Tuna Melt

Quick Recipe   *(Pictured below)*

- 1 can (12 ounces) chunk white tuna packed in water, drained and flaked
- 1-1/2 cups coleslaw mix
- 3 tablespoons sliced green onions
- 3 tablespoons reduced-fat mayonnaise
- 1 tablespoon Dijon mustard
- 1 teaspoon dill weed
- 4 English muffins, split and lightly toasted
- 1/3 cup shredded reduced-fat Cheddar cheese

1. Preheat broiler. Combine tuna, coleslaw mix and green onions in medium bowl. Combine mayonnaise, mustard and dill weed in small bowl. Stir mayonnaise mixture into tuna mixture.

2. Spread tuna mixture onto muffin halves. Place on broiler pan. Broil 4 inches from heat 3 to 4 minutes or until heated through. Sprinkle evenly with cheese. Broil 1 to 2 minutes more or until cheese melts.   *Makes 4 servings*

Nutrients per Serving: 2 Melts

Calories 313	**Fiber** 2g	
Fat 8g (sat 2g)	**Cholesterol** 43mg	
Protein 30g	**Sodium** 882mg	
Carbohydrate 30g		

Exchanges: 2 starch, 3 lean meat

Tuna Melts

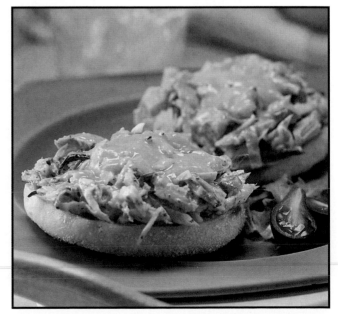

Moroccan Grilled Turkey with Cucumber Yogurt Sauce

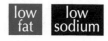

Quick Recipe *(Pictured at right)*

Cucumber Yogurt Sauce (recipe follows)
1 package BUTTERBALL® Fresh Boneless
  Turkey Breast Cutlets
1/3 cup fresh lime juice
2 cloves garlic, minced
1/2 teaspoon salt
1/2 teaspoon curry powder
1/4 teaspoon ground cumin
1/4 teaspoon cayenne pepper
3 large pitas, cut in half*

*Pitas may be filled and folded in half.

Prepare Cucumber Yogurt Sauce. Prepare grill for medium-direct-heat cooking. Lightly spray unheated grill rack with nonstick cooking spray. Combine lime juice, garlic, salt, curry powder, cumin and cayenne pepper in medium bowl. Dip cutlets in lime juice mixture. Place cutlets on rack over medium-hot grill. Grill 5 to 7 minutes on each side or until meat is no longer pink in center. Place turkey and Cucumber Yogurt Sauce in pitas.   *Makes 6 servings*

Cucumber Yogurt Sauce
1 cup fat free yogurt
1/2 cup shredded cucumber
1 teaspoon grated lime peel
1 teaspoon salt
1/2 teaspoon ground cumin

Combine yogurt, cucumber, lime peel, salt and cumin in medium bowl. Chill.

Nutrients per Serving: 1 sandwich (1/2 pita with 1 Turkey Cutlet and 3 tablespoons plus 1 teaspoon Cucumber Yogurt Sauce)

Calories 195	**Fiber** 1g
Fat 2g (sat <1g)	**Cholesterol** 46mg
Protein 23g	**Sodium** 647mg
Carbohydrate 20g	

Exchanges: 1-1/2 starch, 2-1/2 lean meat

Mediterranean Fish Soup

Quick Recipe   *(Pictured on page 128)*

4 ounces uncooked pastina or other small
  pasta
Nonstick cooking spray
3/4 cup chopped onion
2 cloves garlic, minced
1 teaspoon fennel seeds
1 can (14-1/2 ounces) no-salt-added
  stewed tomatoes
1 can (14-1/2 ounces) fat-free reduced-
  sodium chicken broth
1 tablespoon minced fresh parsley
1/2 teaspoon black pepper
1/4 teaspoon ground turmeric
8 ounces firm, white-fleshed fish, cut into
  1-inch pieces
3 ounces small uncooked shrimp, peeled
  and deveined

1. Cook pasta according to package directions, omitting salt. Drain and set aside.

2. Spray large nonstick saucepan with cooking spray. Add onion, garlic and fennel seeds; cook over medium heat 3 minutes or until onion is tender.

3. Stir in tomatoes, chicken broth, parsley, pepper and turmeric. Bring to a boil; reduce heat and simmer 10 minutes. Add fish and cook 1 minute. Add shrimp and cook until shrimp just begin to turn pink and opaque.

4. Divide pasta evenly among 4 bowls; ladle soup over pasta.   *Makes 4 servings*

Nutrients per Serving: 1-1/2 cups Soup with 1/2 cup cooked pasta

Calories 209	**Fiber** 3g
Fat 2g (sat <1g)	**Cholesterol** 59mg
Protein 19g	**Sodium** 111mg
Carbohydrate 28g	

Exchanges: 1-1/2 starch, 1 vegetable, 1-1/2 lean meat

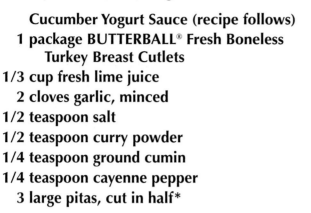

Moroccan Grilled Turkey with Cucumber Yogurt Sauce

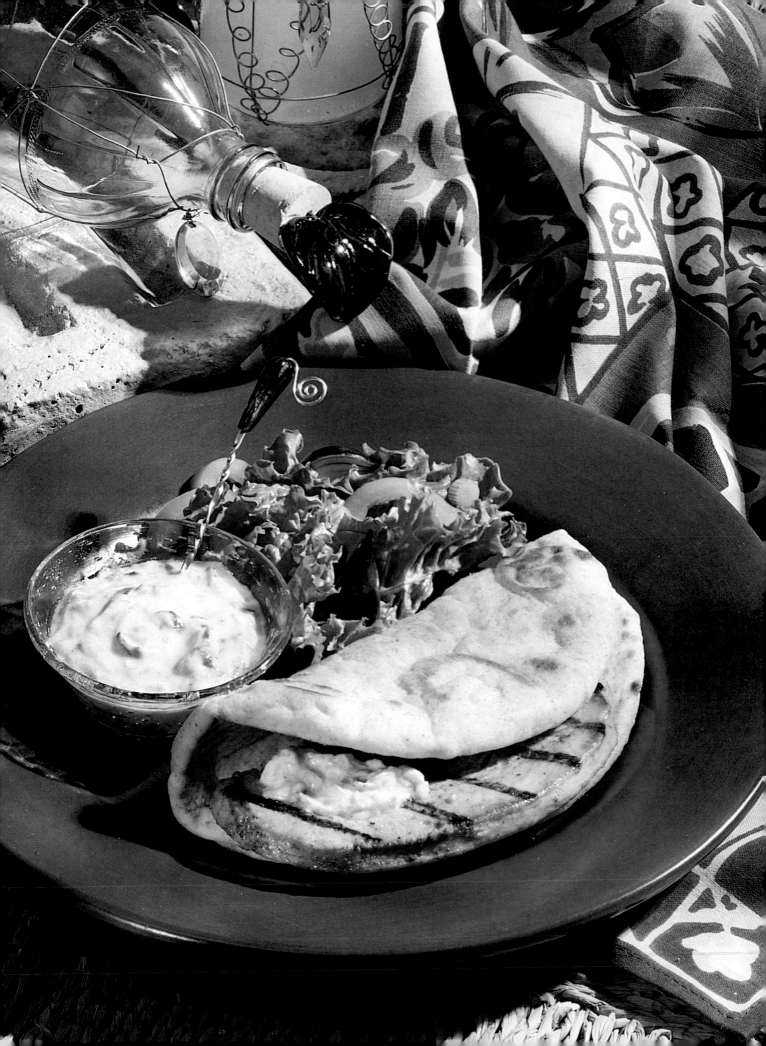

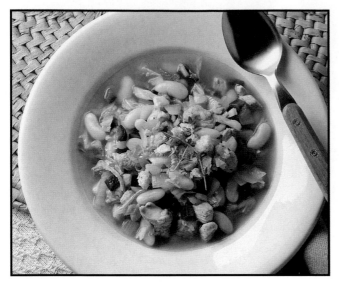

Skillet Chicken Soup

Skillet Chicken Soup
high fiber

Quick Recipe   (Pictured above)

**3/4 pound boneless skinless chicken breasts
     or thighs, cut into 3/4-inch pieces**
1 teaspoon paprika
1/2 teaspoon salt
1/4 teaspoon black pepper
2 teaspoons vegetable oil
1 large onion, chopped
**1 medium red bell pepper, cut into
     1/2-inch pieces**
3 cloves garlic, minced
**1 cup fat-free reduced-sodium chicken
     broth**
**1 can (19 ounces) cannellini beans or
     small white beans, rinsed and drained**
**3 cups sliced savoy, napa or green
     cabbage**
**1/2 cup fat-free herb-flavored croutons,
     slightly crushed**

Toss chicken with paprika, salt and black
pepper in medium bowl until coated. Heat oil
in large, deep nonstick skillet over medium-high
heat until hot. Add chicken, onion, bell pepper
and garlic. Cook until chicken is no longer pink,
stirring frequently. Add broth and beans; bring
to a simmer. Cover and simmer 5 minutes or
until chicken is cooked through. Stir in cabbage;
cover and simmer 3 additional minutes or until

cabbage is wilted. Ladle into 4 shallow bowls; top
with crushed croutons.   *Makes 4 servings*

Nutrients per Serving: 1-1/4 cups Soup with
2 tablespoons crushed croutons

Calories 284	**Fiber** 8g
Fat 5g (sat 1g)	**Cholesterol** 52mg
Protein 28g	**Sodium** 721mg
Carbohydrate 30g	

Exchanges: 1-1/2 starch, 1-1/2 vegetable,
2-1/2 lean meat

❧ ❧ ❧

Tarragon Chicken Salad Sandwiches

Quick Recipe

**1-1/4 pounds boneless skinless chicken
     breasts, cooked**
1 cup thinly sliced celery
**1 cup seedless red or green grapes, cut
     into halves**
1/2 cup raisins
1/2 cup fat-free yogurt
**1/4 cup reduced-fat mayonnaise or salad
     dressing**
**2 tablespoons finely chopped shallots or
     onion**
**1 teaspoon dried tarragon leaves *or*
     2 tablespoons minced fresh tarragon**
1/2 teaspoon salt
1/8 teaspoon white pepper
6 lettuce leaves
6 whole wheat buns, split

Cut chicken into 1/2-inch cubes. Combine
chicken, celery, grapes and raisins in large bowl.
Combine yogurt, mayonnaise, shallots, tarragon,
salt and pepper in small bowl. Mix with chicken
mixture. Divide lettuce and chicken mixture
evenly among buns.   *Makes 6 servings*

Nutrients per Serving: 1 Sandwich (1 bun with 1 cup
Chicken Salad and 1 lettuce leaf)

Calories 353	**Fiber** 4g
Fat 7g (sat 1g)	**Cholesterol** 76mg
Protein 34g	**Sodium** 509mg
Carbohydrate 41g	

Exchanges: 1-1/2 starch, 1/2 fruit, 4 lean meat

Mexican Tortilla Soup

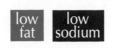

Nonstick cooking spray

2 pounds boneless skinless chicken
    breasts, cut into 1/2-inch strips

4 cups diced carrots

2 cups sliced celery

1 cup chopped green bell pepper

1 cup chopped onion

4 cloves garlic, minced

1 jalapeño pepper,* seeded and sliced

1 teaspoon dried oregano leaves

1/2 teaspoon ground cumin

8 cups fat-free reduced-sodium chicken
    broth

1 large tomato, seeded and chopped

4 to 5 tablespoons lime juice

2 corn tortillas (6 inches), cut into
    1/4-inch strips

Salt (optional)

3 tablespoons finely chopped fresh
    cilantro

*Jalapeño peppers can sting and irritate the skin; wear rubber gloves when handling peppers and do not touch eyes. Wash hands after handling peppers.

1. Preheat oven to 350°F. Spray large nonstick Dutch oven with cooking spray; heat over medium heat. Add chicken; cook and stir about 10 minutes or until browned and no longer pink in center.

2. Add carrots, celery, bell pepper, onion, garlic, jalapeño pepper, oregano and cumin; cook and stir over medium heat 5 minutes. Stir in chicken broth, tomato and lime juice; heat to a boil. Reduce heat to low; cover and simmer 15 to 20 minutes or until carrots are crisp-tender.

3. Meanwhile, spray tortilla strips lightly with cooking spray; sprinkle very lightly with salt, if desired. Place on baking sheet. Bake about 10 minutes or until browned and crisp, stirring occasionally.

4. Stir cilantro into soup. Ladle soup into 8 bowls; top evenly with tortilla strips.

Makes 8 servings

Nutrients per Serving: 1-3/4 cups Soup topped with tortilla strips

Calories 184	**Fiber** 4g
Fat 3g (sat 1g)	**Cholesterol** 58mg
Protein 23g	**Sodium** 132mg
Carbohydrate 16g	

Exchanges: 3 vegetable, 2 lean meat

Rosarita Refried Soup

Quick Recipe

PAM® No-Stick Cooking Spray

1 cup diced onion

1 can (16 ounces) ROSARITA® Traditional
    No-Fat Refried Beans

6 cups fat-free low-sodium chicken broth

1 can (14.5 ounces) HUNT'S® Diced
    Tomatoes in Juice

4 cups baked tortilla chips

1/2 cup shredded reduced-fat Monterey
    Jack cheese

1/4 cup chopped fresh cilantro

1. Spray a large saucepan with PAM® Cooking Spray. Sauté onion over low heat for 5 minutes.

2. Add Rosarita® Beans, broth and Hunt's® Tomatoes; mix well. Cook until heated through.

3. Place *1/3 cup* tortilla chips in *each* bowl. Ladle soup into bowls. Garnish with cheese and cilantro. *Makes 12 (1-cup) servings*

Nutrients per Serving: 1 cup Soup with 1/3 cup tortilla chips and 2 teaspoons cheese

Calories 110	**Fiber** 3g
Fat 2g (sat 1g)	**Cholesterol** 16mg
Protein 8g	**Sodium** 471mg
Carbohydrate 14g	

Exchanges: 1 starch, 1/2 lean meat

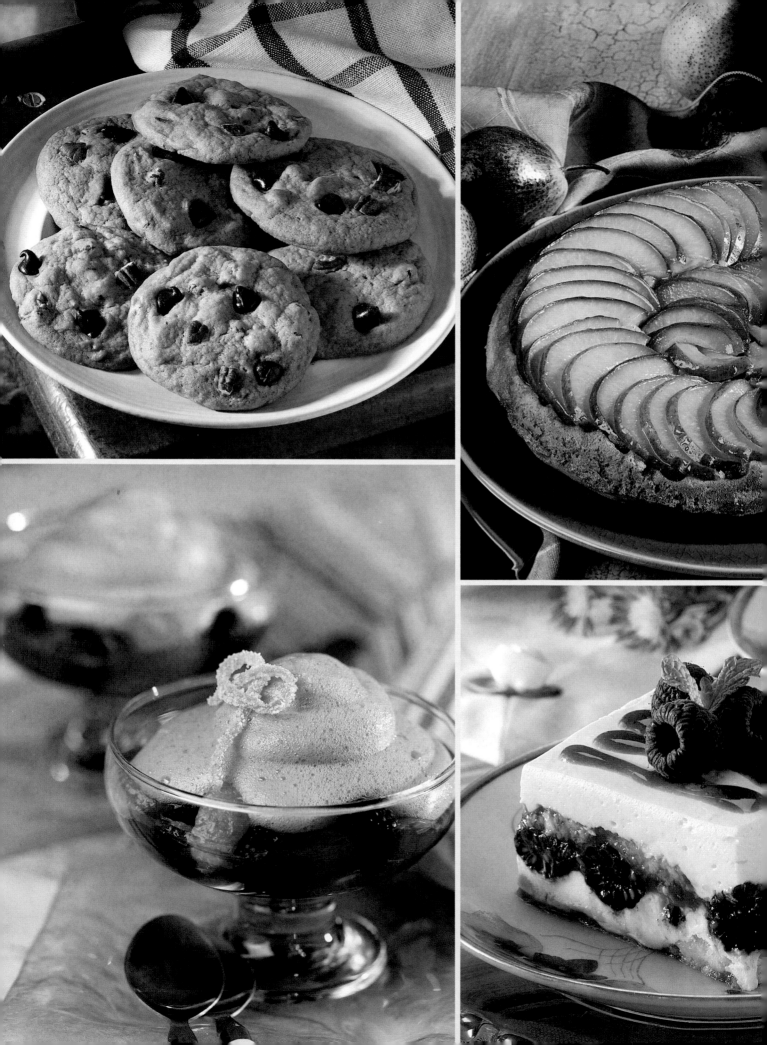

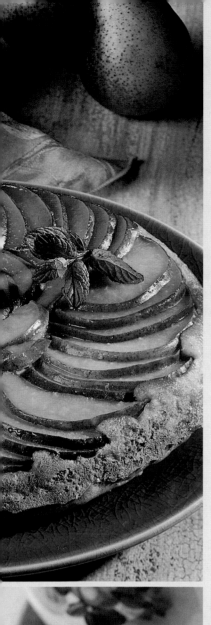

Desserts

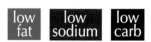

Florida Sunshine Cups

<small>low fat</small> <small>low sodium</small> <small>low carb</small>

(Pictured at left)

3/4 cup boiling water
   1 package (4-serving size) JELL-O® Brand Orange or Lemon Flavor Sugar Free Low Calorie Gelatin
   1 cup cold orange juice
1/2 cup fresh raspberries
   1 can (11 ounces) mandarin orange segments, drained

STIR boiling water into gelatin in large bowl at least 2 minutes until completely dissolved. Stir in cold juice. Refrigerate 1-1/2 hours or until thickened (spoon drawn through leaves definite impression).

MEASURE 3/4 cup thickened gelatin into medium bowl; set aside. Stir fruit into remaining gelatin. Pour into serving bowl or 6 dessert dishes.

BEAT reserved gelatin with electric mixer on high speed until fluffy and about doubled in volume. Spoon over gelatin in bowl or dishes. Garnish as desired.

REFRIGERATE 3 hours or until firm.   *Makes 6 servings*

Nutrients per Serving: 1 Sunshine Cup (1/6 of total recipe)

Calories 50	**Fiber** 1g
Fat <1g (sat <1g)	**Cholesterol** 0mg
Protein 1g	**Sodium** 46mg
Carbohydrate 10g	
Exchanges: 1 fruit	

Clockwise from top left: Chocolate Chip Cookies (page 160), Pear-Ginger Upside-Down Cake (page 170), Lemon Raspberry Tiramisu (page 161) and Florida Sunshine Cups

Fresh Fruit Parfaits

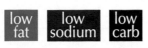

(Pictured at right)

1 cup fresh fruit

3/4 cup boiling water

1 package (4-serving size) JELL-O® Brand
    Sugar Free Low Calorie Gelatin
    Dessert or JELL-O® Brand Gelatin
    Dessert, any flavor

1/2 cup cold water
    Ice cubes

3/4 cup thawed COOL WHIP FREE® or
    COOL WHIP LITE® Whipped Topping

DIVIDE fruit among 6 parfait glasses.

STIR boiling water into gelatin in medium bowl at least 2 minutes until completely dissolved. Mix cold water and ice cubes to make 1-1/4 cups. Add to gelatin, stirring until slightly thickened. Remove any remaining ice. Measure 3/4 cup of the gelatin; pour into parfait glasses. Refrigerate 1 hour or until set but not firm (gelatin should stick to finger when touched and should mound).

STIR whipped topping into remaining gelatin with wire whisk until smooth. Spoon over gelatin in glasses.

REFRIGERATE 1 hour or until firm. Garnish as desired.   *Makes 6 servings*

Nutrients per Serving: 1 Parfait (1/6 of total recipe), made with 1/2 cup *each* blueberries and strawberries, JELL-O® Brand Sugar Free Low Calorie Gelatin Dessert, and COOL WHIP FREE®

Calories 46	**Fiber** 1g
Fat <1g (sat <1g)	**Cholesterol** 0mg
Protein 1g	**Sodium** 38mg
Carbohydrate 9g	

Exchanges: 1 fruit

Apple-Cranberry Crescent Cookies

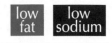

1-1/4 cups chopped apples

1/2 cup dried cranberries

1/2 cup reduced-fat sour cream

1/4 cup cholesterol-free egg substitute

1/4 cup margarine or butter, melted

3 tablespoons sugar, divided

1 package rapid-rise active dry yeast

1 teaspoon vanilla extract

2 cups all-purpose flour

1 teaspoon ground cinnamon

1 tablespoon 2% milk

1. Preheat oven to 350°F. Lightly coat cookie sheet with nonstick cooking spray.

2. Place apples and cranberries in food processor or blender; pulse to finely chop. Set aside.

3. Combine sour cream, egg substitute, margarine and 2 tablespoons sugar in medium bowl. Add yeast and vanilla. Add flour; stir to form ball. Turn dough out onto lightly floured work surface. Knead 1 minute. Cover with plastic wrap; allow to stand 10 minutes.

4. Divide dough into thirds. Roll one portion into 12-inch circle. Spread with 1/3 apple mixture (about 1/4 cup). Cut dough to make 8 wedges. Roll up each wedge, beginning at outside edge. Place on prepared cookie sheet; turn ends of cookies to form crescents. Repeat with remaining dough and apple mixture.

5. Combine remaining 1 tablespoon sugar and cinnamon in small bowl. Lightly brush cookies with milk; sprinkle evenly with sugar-cinnamon mixture. Bake cookies 18 to 20 minutes or until lightly browned.   *Makes 2 dozen cookies*

Nutrients per Serving: 1 Cookie

Calories 82	**Fiber** 1g
Fat 2g (sat 1g)	**Cholesterol** 2mg
Protein 2g	**Sodium** 31mg
Carbohydrate 13g	

Exchanges: 1 starch

Fresh Fruit Parfaits

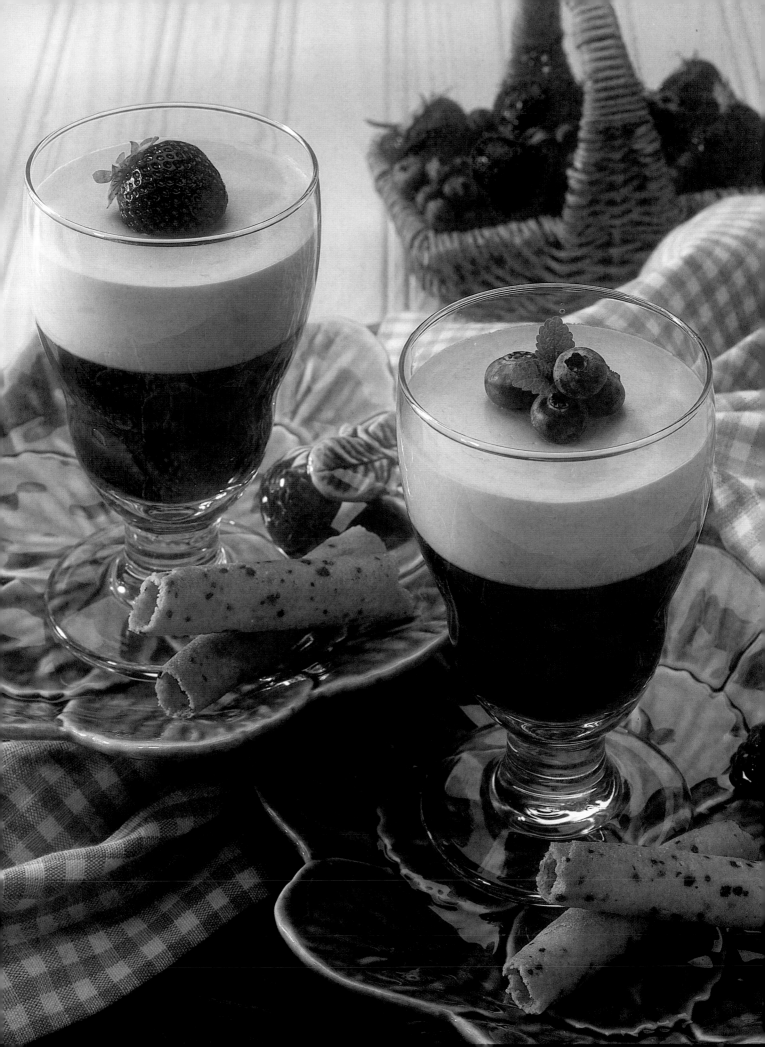

Key Lime Tarts

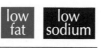

(Pictured at right)

- 3/4 cup fat-free milk
- 6 tablespoons fresh lime juice
- 2 tablespoons cornstarch
- 1/2 cup cholesterol-free egg substitute
- 1/2 cup reduced-fat sour cream
- 12 packets sugar substitute* *or* equivalent of 1/2 cup sugar
- 4 sheets phyllo dough**
  Butter-flavored nonstick cooking spray
- 3/4 cup thawed frozen fat-free nondairy whipped topping
  Fresh raspberries and lime slices (optional)

This recipe was tested with Equal® sweetener.

**Cover with damp kitchen towel to prevent dough from drying out.*

1. Combine milk, lime juice and cornstarch in medium saucepan. Cook over medium heat 2 to 3 minutes, stirring constantly until thick. Remove from heat. Add egg substitute; whisk constantly for 30 seconds to allow egg substitute to cook. Stir in sour cream and sugar substitute; cover and refrigerate until cool.

2. Preheat oven to 350°F. Spray 8 (2-1/2-inch) muffin cups with cooking spray; set aside. Place 1 sheet of phyllo dough on cutting board; spray with cooking spray. Top with second sheet of phyllo dough; spray with cooking spray. Top with third sheet of phyllo dough; spray with cooking spray. Top with last sheet; spray with cooking spray.

3. Cut stack of phyllo dough into 8 squares. Gently fit each stacked square into prepared muffin cup; press firmly against bottom and side. Bake 8 to 10 minutes or until golden brown. Carefully remove from muffin cups; cool on wire rack. Divide lime mixture evenly among phyllo cups; top evenly with whipped topping. Garnish with fresh raspberries and lime slices, if desired. *Makes 8 servings*

Nutrients per Serving: 1 Tart

Calories 82	**Fiber** <1g
Fat 1g (sat <1g)	**Cholesterol** 5mg
Protein 3g	**Sodium** 88mg
Carbohydrate 13g	

Exchanges: 1 starch

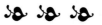

Lemon Mousse with Raspberry Sauce

- 1-1/2 cups boiling water
- 1 package (8-serving size) *or* 2 packages (4-serving size each) JELL-O® Brand Lemon Flavor Sugar Free Low Calorie Gelatin
- 2 teaspoons grated lemon peel
- 1 cup cold apple juice
  Ice cubes
- 1 tub (8 ounces) COOL WHIP FREE® Whipped Topping, thawed
- 1 package (10 ounces) frozen raspberries or strawberries, thawed, puréed in blender

STIR boiling water into gelatin and lemon peel in large bowl at least 2 minutes until gelatin is completely dissolved. Mix apple juice and ice to measure 1-3/4 cups. Add to gelatin, stirring until slightly thickened. Remove any remaining ice.

STIR in whipped topping with wire whisk. Pour into serving bowl or 10 dessert dishes.

REFRIGERATE 4 hours or until firm. Serve with raspberry sauce. *Makes 10 servings*

Nutrients per Serving: about 1/2 cup Lemon Mousse with about 1-1/4 tablespoons Rasperry Sauce

Calories 80	**Fiber** 2g
Fat 2g (sat 1g)	**Cholesterol** 0mg
Protein 2g	**Sodium** 60mg
Carbohydrate 15g	

Exchanges: 1 starch

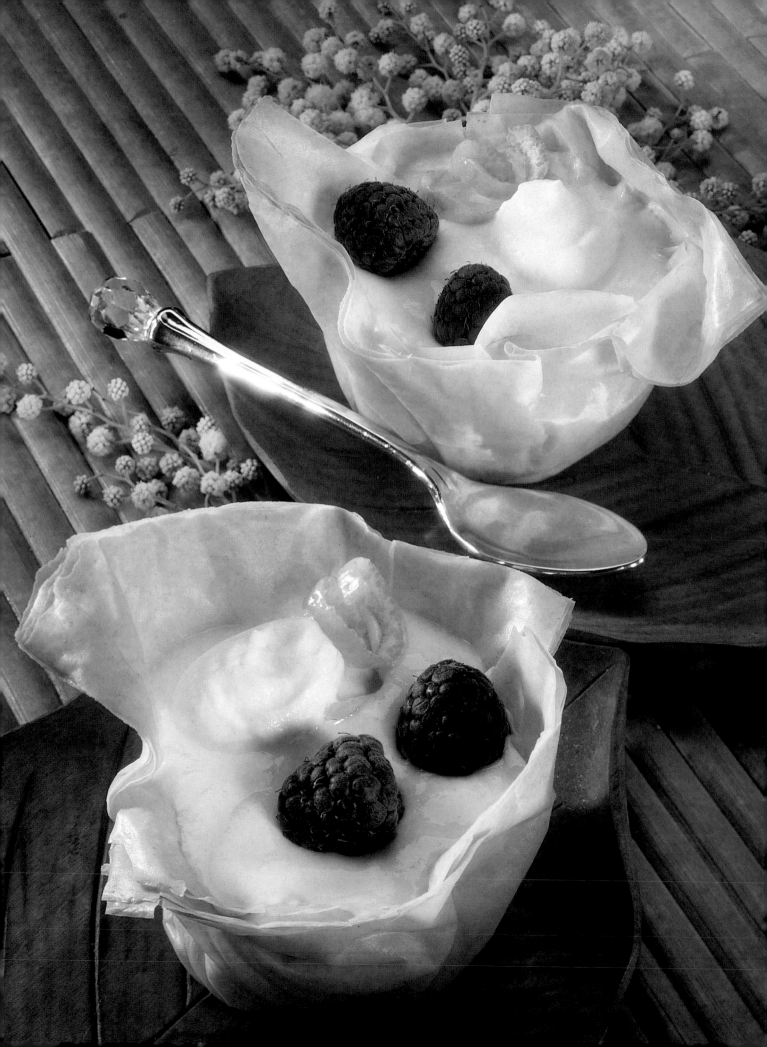

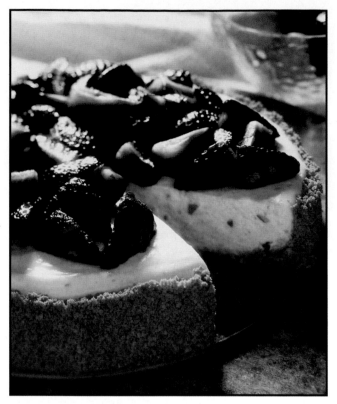

*Lime Cheesecake with
Strawberries and Fresh Mint*

Lime Cheesecake with Strawberries and Fresh Mint

(Pictured above)

**9 whole low-fat honey graham crackers,
  broken into small pieces**

5 tablespoons reduced-fat margarine

**2 packages (8 ounces each) reduced-fat
  cream cheese**

1 package (8 ounces) fat-free cream cheese

**1 container (6 ounces) plain fat-free
  yogurt**

2/3 cup powdered sugar

1/4 cup lime juice

1/3 cup sugar substitute,* divided

2 teaspoons lime peel

1-1/2 teaspoons vanilla extract

3 cups fresh strawberries, quartered

2 tablespoons finely chopped mint leaves

* This recipe was tested with Splenda® Granular.

158 **Desserts**

1. Preheat oven to 350°F. Coat 9-inch springform baking pan with nonstick cooking spray; set aside.

2. Place graham cracker pieces and margarine in food processor or blender; pulse until coarse in texture.

3. Gently press crumb mixture onto bottom and 1/2 inch up side of pan. Bake 8 to 10 minutes or until lightly browned; cool completely on wire rack.

4. Beat cream cheese, yogurt, powdered sugar, lime juice, 1/4 cup sugar substitute, lime peel and vanilla in large bowl with electric mixer at high speed until smooth. Pour into cooled pie crust.

5. Cover with plastic wrap; freeze 2 hours or refrigerate overnight.

6. Combine strawberries, remaining sugar substitute and mint in medium bowl 30 minutes before serving; set aside.

7. Just before serving, spoon strawberry mixture evenly over cheesecake.　　*Makes 12 servings*

Nutrients per Serving: 1 slice Cheesecake with topping (1/12 of total recipe)

Calories 151	**Fiber** 1g
Fat 7g (sat 3g)	**Cholesterol** 14mg
Protein 5g	**Sodium** 224mg
Carbohydrate 18g	

Exchanges: 1/2 fruit, 1 milk, 1 fat

Tip

Three medium-size limes yield about 1/4 cup lime juice and 4-1/2 teaspoons grated lime peel. Get the most juice from the limes by bringing them to room temperature and rolling them around on the counter while pressing down with the palm of your hand. Grate the peel before you squeeze the juice. Scrub the limes in warm, soapy water. Then, using a box-shaped grater, a zester or a vegetable peeler, remove the peel or "zest." Be sure to remove only the colored part of the peel and not the bitter white pith underneath.

Baked Pear Dessert

low fat **low sodium** **cooking for 1 or 2**

(Pictured below)

2 tablespoons dried cranberries or raisins

1 tablespoon toasted sliced almonds

1/8 teaspoon ground cinnamon

1/3 cup unsweetened apple cider or apple juice, divided

1 medium unpeeled pear (6 ounces), cut in half lengthwise and cored

1/2 cup vanilla low-fat no-sugar-added frozen ice cream or frozen yogurt

1. Preheat oven to 350°F. Combine cranberries, almonds, cinnamon and 1 teaspoon cider in small bowl.

2. Place pear halves, cut sides up, in small baking dish. Evenly mound almond mixture on top of pear halves. Pour remaining cider into dish. Cover with foil.

3. Bake pear halves 35 to 40 minutes or until pears are soft, spooning cider in dish over pears once or twice during baking. Serve warm with ice cream. *Makes 2 servings*

Nutrients per Serving: 1 topped pear half with 1/4 cup ice cream

Calories 87	**Fiber** 1g
Fat 2g (sat <1g)	**Cholesterol** 3mg
Protein 1g	**Sodium** 13mg
Carbohydrate 16g	

Exchanges: 1 fruit, 1/2 fat

Baked Pear Dessert

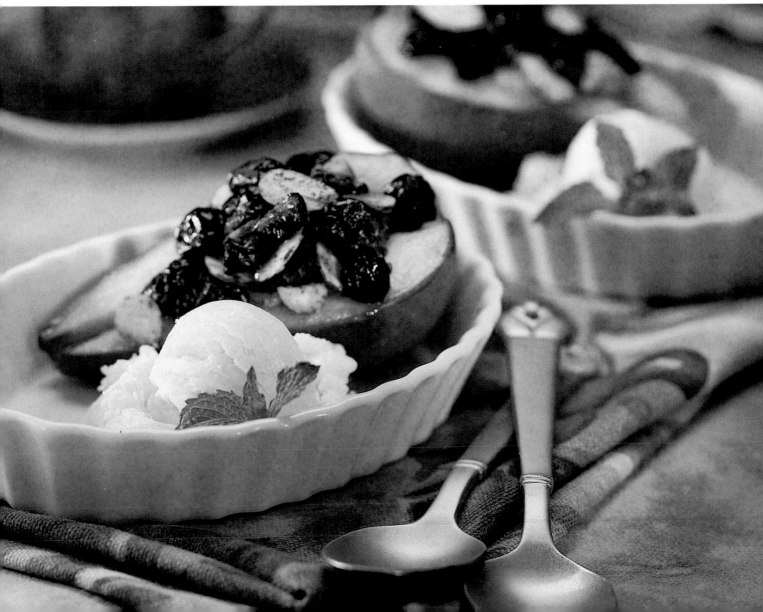

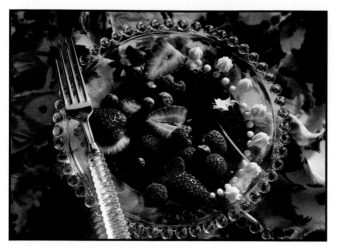

Fantasy in Berries

Fantasy in Berries

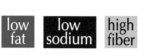

Quick Recipe   *(Pictured above)*

>   1 bag (12 ounces) frozen unsweetened
>   raspberries, thawed
> 1/4 cup plus 2 tablespoons sugar, divided
>   1 tablespoon fresh lemon juice
>   2 cups sliced fresh strawberries
>   1 cup fresh raspberries
>   1 cup fresh blueberries
>   1 cup reduced-fat ricotta cheese
>   1 teaspoon vanilla extract
> 1/4 teaspoon almond extract

1. Place thawed frozen raspberries, 1/4 cup sugar and lemon juice in blender or food processor; blend until smooth. Pour through strainer to remove seeds. Spoon 3 tablespoons raspberry sauce onto each of 8 plates. Tilt each plate, rotating to spread raspberry sauce over plate. Arrange 1/4 cup sliced strawberries and 2 tablespoons each fresh raspberries and blueberries on top of sauce on each plate.

2. Place cheese, remaining 2 tablespoons sugar and vanilla and almond extracts in clean blender or food processor; blend until smooth and satiny. Spoon cheese mixture into pastry bag; pipe onto berries, about 2 tablespoons per serving.   *Makes 8 servings*

Nutrients per Serving: 1/8 of total recipe

Calories 104	**Fiber** 5g
Fat 1g (sat <1g)	**Cholesterol** 4mg
Protein 4g	**Sodium** 25mg
Carbohydrate 21g	

Exchanges: 1-1/2 fruit, 1/2 lean meat

ᕶᕘ ᕶᕘ ᕶᕘ

Chocolate Chip Cookies

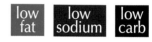

(Pictured on page 152)

>   8 tablespoons margarine, softened
> 1-1/2 cups packed light brown sugar
>   2 egg whites
>   1 teaspoon vanilla extract
> 2-1/2 cups all-purpose flour
> 1-1/2 teaspoons baking soda
>   1/2 teaspoon salt
>   1/3 cup fat-free milk
>   3/4 cup (4 ounces) semisweet chocolate
>   chips
>   1/2 cup chopped pecans or walnuts
>   (optional)

1. Preheat oven to 350°F. Spray cookie sheets with nonstick cooking spray.

2. Beat margarine and brown sugar in large bowl until fluffy. Beat in egg whites and vanilla. Combine flour, baking soda and salt in medium bowl. Add flour mixture to margarine mixture alternately with milk, ending with flour mixture. Stir in chocolate chips and pecans, if desired.

3. Drop dough by slightly rounded tablespoonfuls onto prepared cookie sheets. Bake about 10 minutes or until lightly browned. Cool on wire racks.

Makes about 6 dozen cookies

Nutrients per Serving: 1 Cookie

Calories 56	**Fiber** 0g
Fat 2g (sat 0g)	**Cholesterol** 0mg
Protein 1g	**Sodium** 61mg
Carbohydrate 10g	

Exchanges: 1/2 starch, 1/2 fat

Lemon Raspberry Tiramisu

(Pictured on page 152)

2 packages (8 ounces each) fat-free cream cheese, softened

6 packets sugar substitute* *or* equivalent of 1/4 cup sugar

1 teaspoon vanilla extract

1/3 cup water

1 package (4-serving size) sugar-free lemon-flavored gelatin

2 cups thawed frozen fat-free nondairy whipped topping

1/2 cup all-fruit red raspberry preserves

1/4 cup water

2 tablespoons marsala wine (optional)

2 packages (3 ounces each) ladyfingers

1 pint fresh raspberries or frozen unsweetened raspberries, thawed

*This recipe was tested with Equal® sweetener.

1. Combine cream cheese, sugar substitute and vanilla in large bowl. Beat with electric mixer at high speed until smooth; set aside. Combine water and gelatin in small microwavable bowl; microwave at HIGH 30 seconds to 1 minute or until water is boiling and gelatin is dissolved. Cool slightly. Add gelatin mixture to cheese mixture; beat 1 minute. Add whipped topping; beat 1 minute more, scraping side of bowl. Set aside.

2. Whisk together preserves, water and marsala, if desired, in small bowl until well blended. Reserve 2 tablespoons of preserves mixture; set aside. Spread 1/3 cup preserves mixture evenly over bottom of 11×7-inch glass baking dish.

3. Split ladyfingers in half; place half in bottom of baking dish. Spread half of cheese mixture evenly over ladyfingers; sprinkle 1 cup raspberries evenly over cheese mixture. Top with remaining ladyfingers; spread remaining preserves mixture over ladyfingers. Top with remaining cheese mixture. Cover; refrigerate at least 2 hours. Drizzle with reserved 2 tablespoons preserves mixture and sprinkle with remaining raspberries before serving. Garnish as desired.

Makes 12 servings

Nutrients per Serving: 1 slice Tiramisu (1/12 of total recipe)

Calories 158	**Fiber** 1g
Fat 1g (sat <1g)	**Cholesterol** 52mg
Protein 7g	**Sodium** 272mg
Carbohydrate 26g	

Exchanges: 2 starch

ᔓ ᔓ ᔓ

Cherry Cocoa Cake

1 cup water

1/2 cup unsweetened cocoa powder

1/2 cup margarine

2 cups all-purpose flour

1-3/4 cups sugar

1/2 cup low-fat cherry yogurt

1 egg, slightly beaten

1 teaspoon baking soda

1 teaspoon vanilla extract

1/2 teaspoon salt

1 tablespoon powdered sugar

In large saucepan, combine water, cocoa and margarine. Cook over medium heat, stirring frequently, until mixture comes to a full boil. Remove from heat; stir in flour and sugar. Add yogurt, egg, baking soda, vanilla and salt; mix thoroughly.

Pour batter into 15-1/2×10-inch baking pan coated with nonstick cooking spray. Bake at 375°F for 20 to 25 minutes or until wooden pick inserted into center comes out clean. Cool in pan on wire rack. Sprinkle powdered sugar evenly over top. Cut into 32 squares.

Makes 32 servings

Favorite recipe from **North Dakota Wheat Commission**

Nutrients per Serving: 1 Cake square

Calories 105	**Fiber** <1g
Fat 3g (sat 1g)	**Cholesterol** 7mg
Protein 1g	**Sodium** 113mg
Carbohydrate 18g	

Exchanges: 1 starch, 1/2 fat

Creamy Strawberry-Orange Pops

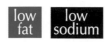 low fat low sodium

(Pictured at right)

1 container (8 ounces) strawberry-flavored yogurt with aspartame sweetener

3/4 cup orange juice

2 teaspoons vanilla extract

2 cups frozen whole strawberries

1 packet sugar substitute* *or* equivalent of 2 teaspoons sugar

6 paper cups (7 ounces)

6 wooden sticks

*This recipe was tested with Equal® sweetener.

1. Combine yogurt, orange juice and vanilla in food processor or blender. Cover and blend until smooth.

2. Add frozen strawberries and sugar substitute. Blend until smooth. Pour into 6 paper cups, filling each about 3/4 full. Place in freezer for 1 hour. Insert wooden stick into center of each. Freeze completely. Peel cup off each to serve.

Makes 6 servings

Nutrients per Serving: 1 Pop

Calories 97	**Fiber** 1g
Fat <1g (sat <1g)	**Cholesterol** 1mg
Protein 6g	**Sodium** 139mg
Carbohydrate 17g	

Exchanges: 1 fruit, 1/2 milk

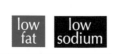

Strawberry Delights

low fat low sodium

Quick Recipe

2 cups low-fat strawberry ice cream

1 cup sliced fresh strawberries

2/3 cup cold fat-free milk

1/4 cup cold orange juice

1/8 teaspoon ground cinnamon

1. Place ice cream, strawberries, milk, orange juice and cinnamon in blender or food processor. Blend at high speed until smooth.

2. Pour into 4 glasses. Garnish with additional fruit and mint leaves, if desired.

Makes 4 servings

Nutrients per Serving: 1 cup Strawberry Delight (without fruit garnish)

Calories 133	**Fiber** 1g
Fat 2g (sat 1g)	**Cholesterol** 11mg
Protein 5g	**Sodium** 62mg
Carbohydrate 25g	

Exchanges: 1 starch, 1/2 fruit, 1/2 fat

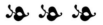

Berries with Banana Cream

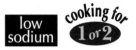 low sodium cooking for 1 or 2

Quick Recipe

1/3 cup reduced-fat sour cream

1/2 small ripe banana, cut into chunks

1 tablespoon frozen orange juice concentrate

2 cups sliced strawberries, blueberries, raspberries or a combination

Ground cinnamon or nutmeg

1. Combine sour cream, banana and juice concentrate in blender. Cover and blend until smooth.

2. Place berries in two serving dishes. Top with sour cream mixture. Sprinkle with cinnamon.

Makes 2 servings

Nutrients per Serving: 1 cup Berries with about 3 tablespoons sour cream mixture

Calories 135	**Fiber** 4g
Fat 4g (sat 3g)	**Cholesterol** 13mg
Protein 4g	**Sodium** 29mg
Carbohydrate 23g	

Exchanges: 1-1/2 fruit, 1 fat

Creamy Strawberry-Orange Pops

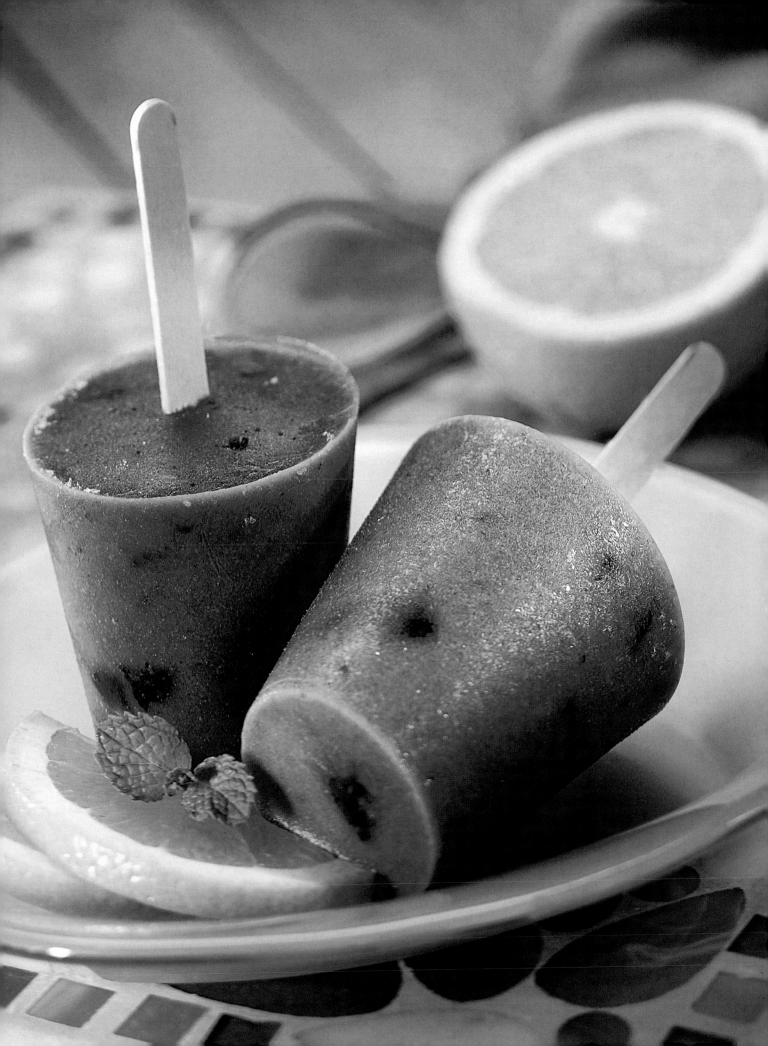

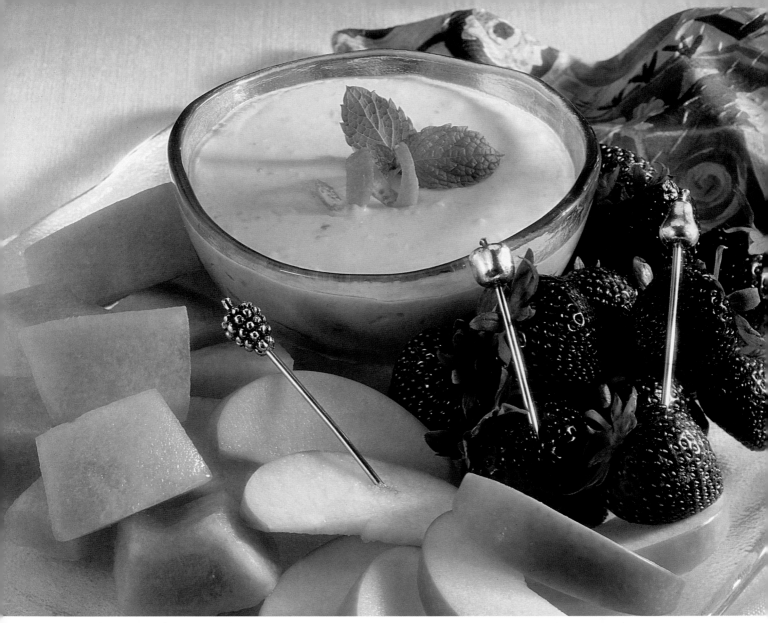

Dreamy Orange Cheesecake Dip

Dreamy Orange Cheesecake Dip

Quick Recipe   *(Pictured above)*

1 package (8 ounces) reduced-fat cream cheese, softened

1/2 cup orange marmalade

1/2 teaspoon vanilla extract

   Grated orange peel (optional)

   Mint leaves (optional)

2 cups whole strawberries

2 cups cantaloupe chunks

2 cups apple slices

1. Combine cream cheese, marmalade and vanilla in small bowl; mix well. Garnish with orange zest and mint leaves, if desired.

2. Serve with fruit dippers.

Makes 12 servings

Note: Dip may be prepared ahead of time. Store, covered, in refrigerator for up to 2 days.

Nutrients per Serving: 2 tablespoons Dip with 1/2 cup fruit

Calories 102	**Fiber** 2g
Fat 4g (sat 2g)	**Cholesterol** 7mg
Protein 3g	**Sodium** 111mg
Carbohydrate 18g	

Exchanges: 1 fruit, 1/2 lean meat, 1/2 fat

Frosted Sugar Cookies

low fat **low sodium**

10 tablespoons margarine, softened
1 cup sugar
2 egg whites
1 teaspoon vanilla extract
2 cups all-purpose flour
1 teaspoon baking powder
1/2 teaspoon salt
Vanilla Frosting (recipe follows)
Ground nutmeg or cinnamon

1. Preheat oven to 375°F. Spray cookie sheets with nonstick cooking spray.

2. Beat margarine and sugar in large bowl with electric mixer at medium speed until fluffy. Beat in egg whites and vanilla.

3. Combine flour, baking powder and salt in medium bowl. Add flour mixture to margarine mixture; mix well. Refrigerate 3 to 4 hours.

4. Roll out dough on generously floured surface to 1/4-inch thickness (dough will be soft). Cut decorative shapes out of dough with 2-inch cookie cutters and place on prepared cookie sheets.

5. Bake 8 to 10 minutes or until cookies turn golden brown. Remove from cookie sheets to wire racks; cool completely. Meanwhile, prepare Vanilla Frosting.

6. Frost cookies; sprinkle with nutmeg or cinnamon.   *Makes 7 dozen cookies*

Vanilla Frosting

2 cups powdered sugar
2 to 3 tablespoons fat-free milk, divided
1 teaspoon vanilla extract

Mix powdered sugar, 2 tablespoons milk and vanilla in medium bowl with fork. Add additional 1 tablespoon milk until desired spreading consistency is reached.
Makes about 1/2 cup frosting

Hint: Keep the cookie dough from sticking to the cookie cutter by simply dipping the cutter in flour before each use.

Nutrients per Serving: 1 Cookie

Calories 44	**Fiber** 0g
Fat 1g (sat 0g)	**Cholesterol** 0mg
Protein 0g	**Sodium** 34mg
Carbohydrate 7g	

Exchanges: 1/2 starch

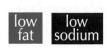

Quick Chocolate Chip Cookie Cakes

low fat **low sodium**

Quick Recipe

1 package (18.25 ounces) reduced-fat yellow cake mix
1/2 cup cholesterol-free egg substitute
1/4 cup vegetable oil
1/4 cup reduced-fat sour cream
2 cups uncooked old-fashioned oats
1/2 cup reduced-fat semisweet chocolate chips

1. Preheat oven to 350°F. Lightly coat cookie sheets with nonstick cooking spray; set aside.

2. Combine cake mix, egg substitute, oil and sour cream in medium bowl. Add oats and chocolate chips.

3. Drop dough by even teaspoonfuls onto prepared cookie sheets.

4. Bake 12 minutes or until lightly browned. Remove to wire racks and cool completely.
Makes 4 dozen cookies

Nutrients per Serving: 1 Cookie Cake

Calories 79	**Fiber** <1g
Fat 3g (sat 1g)	**Cholesterol** <1mg
Protein 1g	**Sodium** 74mg
Carbohydrate 13g	

Exchanges: 1 starch

Lemon-Cranberry Bars

low fat

(Pictured at right)

1/2 cup frozen lemonade concentrate, thawed

1/2 cup spoonable sugar substitute*

1/4 cup margarine

1 egg

1-1/2 cups all-purpose flour

2 teaspoons grated lemon peel

1/2 teaspoon baking soda

1/2 teaspoon salt

1/2 cup dried cranberries

This recipe was tested with Equal® Spoonful™.

1. Preheat oven to 375°F. Lightly coat 8-inch square baking pan with nonstick cooking spray; set aside.

2. Combine lemonade concentrate, sugar substitute, margarine and egg in medium bowl; mix well.

3. Add flour, lemon peel, baking soda and salt; stir well.

4. Stir in cranberries; spoon into prepared pan.

5. Bake 20 minutes or until light brown. Cool completely in pan on wire rack. Cut into 16 squares. *Makes 16 bars*

Nutrients per Serving: 1 Bar (1/16 of total recipe)

Calories 104	**Fiber** <1g
Fat 3g (sat 1g)	**Cholesterol** 13mg
Protein 3g	**Sodium** 150mg
Carbohydrate 15g	

Exchanges: 1 starch, 1/2 fat

Raspberry Swirl Cheesecake

low fat

2 tablespoons vanilla wafer cookie crumbs

2 containers (12 ounces each) fat-free cream cheese

2/3 cup sugar

2 eggs

2 tablespoons cornstarch

2 teaspoons vanilla extract

1 cup reduced-fat sour cream

1 pint (2 cups) raspberries, divided

Mint sprigs for garnish

1. Preheat oven to 400°F. Coat bottom and 1 inch up side of 9-inch springform pan with nonstick cooking spray; firmly press cookie crumbs onto coated bottom and side.

2. Beat cream cheese in large bowl with electric mixer until fluffy. Beat in sugar. Add eggs, cornstarch and vanilla; beat until smooth. Stir in sour cream until well combined. Pour batter into prepared pan.

3. Place 1 cup raspberries in food processor or blender; process until smooth. Strain purée; discard seeds. Spoon purée onto cheesecake; swirl into batter with knife.

4. Bake 45 to 50 minutes or until cheesecake is set around edge but slightly soft in center. Turn off oven; let cheesecake cool in oven about 3 hours, with oven door slightly opened.

5. Refrigerate cheesecake overnight. Remove side of pan; place cheesecake on serving plate. Garnish with remaining 1 cup raspberries and mint sprigs. *Makes 14 servings*

Nutrients per Serving: 1 slice Cheesecake (1/14 of total recipe)

Calories 136	**Fiber** <1g
Fat 3g (sat <1g)	**Cholesterol** 46mg
Protein 9g	**Sodium** 326mg
Carbohydrate 17g	

Exchanges: 1 starch, 1 lean meat

Lemon-Cranberry Bars

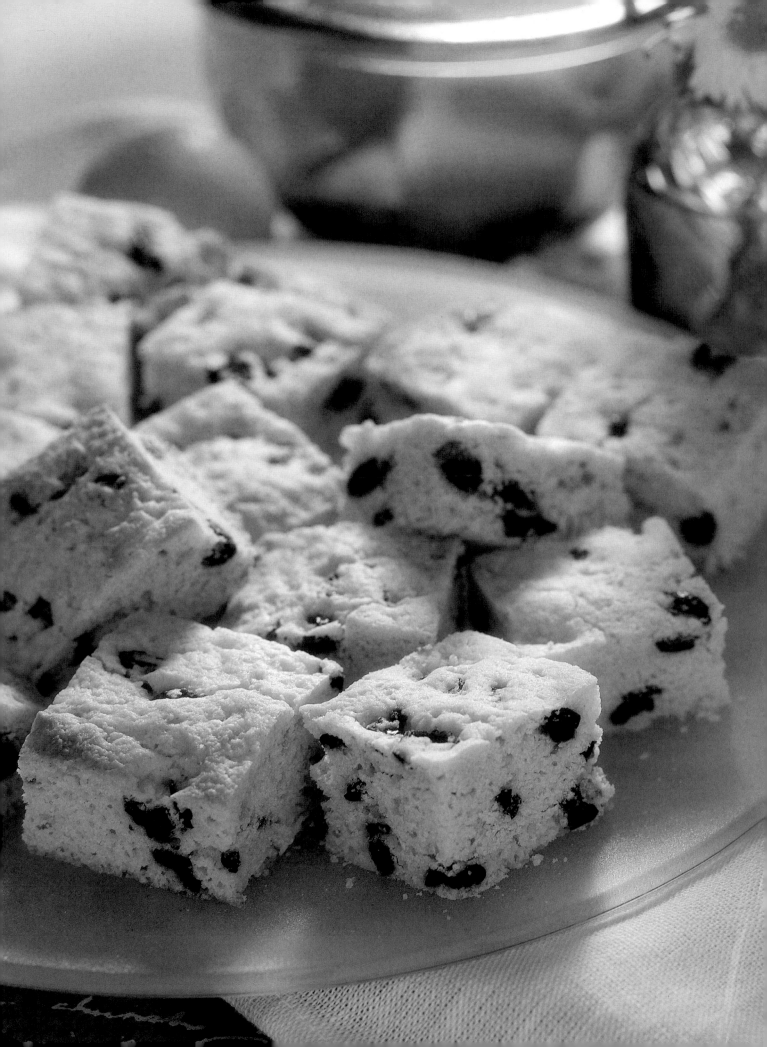

Peach Melba Dessert

(Pictured at right)

1-1/2 cups boiling water, divided

2 packages (4-serving size each) JELL-O® Brand Raspberry Flavor Sugar Free Low Calorie Gelatin Dessert or JELL-O® Brand Raspberry Flavor Gelatin Dessert, divided

1 container (8 ounces) BREYERS® Vanilla Lowfat Yogurt

1 cup raspberries, divided

1 can (8 ounces) peach slices in juice, undrained

Cold water

STIR 3/4 cup boiling water into 1 package of gelatin in large bowl at least 2 minutes until completely dissolved. Refrigerate about 30 minutes or until slightly thickened (consistency of unbeaten egg whites). Stir in yogurt and 1/2 cup raspberries. Pour gelatin mixture into serving bowl. Refrigerate about 2 hours or until set but not firm (gelatin should stick to finger when touched and should mound).

MEANWHILE, drain peaches, reserving juice. Add cold water to reserved juice to make 1 cup; set aside. Stir remaining 3/4 cup boiling water into remaining package gelatin in large bowl at least 2 minutes until completely dissolved. Stir in measured juice and water. Refrigerate about 1 hour or until slightly thickened (consistency of unbeaten egg whites).

RESERVE several peach slices for garnish; chop remaining peaches. Stir chopped peaches into slightly thickened gelatin. Spoon over gelatin layer in bowl. Refrigerate 3 hours or until firm. Top with reserved peach slices and raspberries.

Makes 8 servings

Nutrients per Serving: 1/2 cup Peach Melba Dessert (made with JELL-O® Brand Raspberry Flavor Sugar Free Low Calorie Gelatin Dessert)

Calories 64	**Fiber** 1g
Fat 1g (sat <1g)	**Cholesterol** 2mg
Protein 3g	**Sodium** 81mg
Carbohydrate 11g	

Exchanges: 1 starch

Cheesy Cherry Turnovers

Butter-flavored nonstick cooking spray

1 package (8 ounces) reduced-fat cream cheese, softened

1 cup low-fat (1%) cottage cheese

1/2 cup sugar, divided

1 teaspoon vanilla extract

1 can (16-1/2 ounces) dark sweet pitted cherries, rinsed and drained

8 sheets frozen phyllo dough, thawed

1 cup whole wheat bread crumbs

1 teaspoon ground cinnamon

1. Preheat oven to 350°F. Spray baking sheet with cooking spray; set aside.

2. Combine cream cheese, cottage cheese, 1/4 cup sugar and vanilla in medium bowl with electric mixer. Beat at medium speed until well blended. Stir in cherries.

3. Spray 1 phyllo dough sheet with cooking spray; fold sheet lengthwise in half to form rectangle. Sprinkle with 2 tablespoons bread crumbs. Drop 1/3-cupful cheese mixture onto upper left corner of sheet. Fold right corner over mixture to form triangle. Continue folding triangle, as you would fold a flag, until end of dough is reached. Repeat with remaining ingredients.

4. Place turnovers on prepared baking sheet. Combine remaining 1/4 cup sugar with cinnamon. Evenly sprinkle turnovers with sugar mixture. Bake 12 to 15 minutes or until turnovers are crisp and golden brown. Serve warm or cold.

Makes 8 servings

Nutrients per Serving: 1 Turnover

Calories 170	**Fiber** 1g
Fat 6g (sat 3g)	**Cholesterol** 11mg
Protein 8g	**Sodium** 314mg
Carbohydrate 24g	

Exchanges: 1 starch, 1/2 fruit, 1/2 lean meat, 1 fat

Peach Melba Dessert

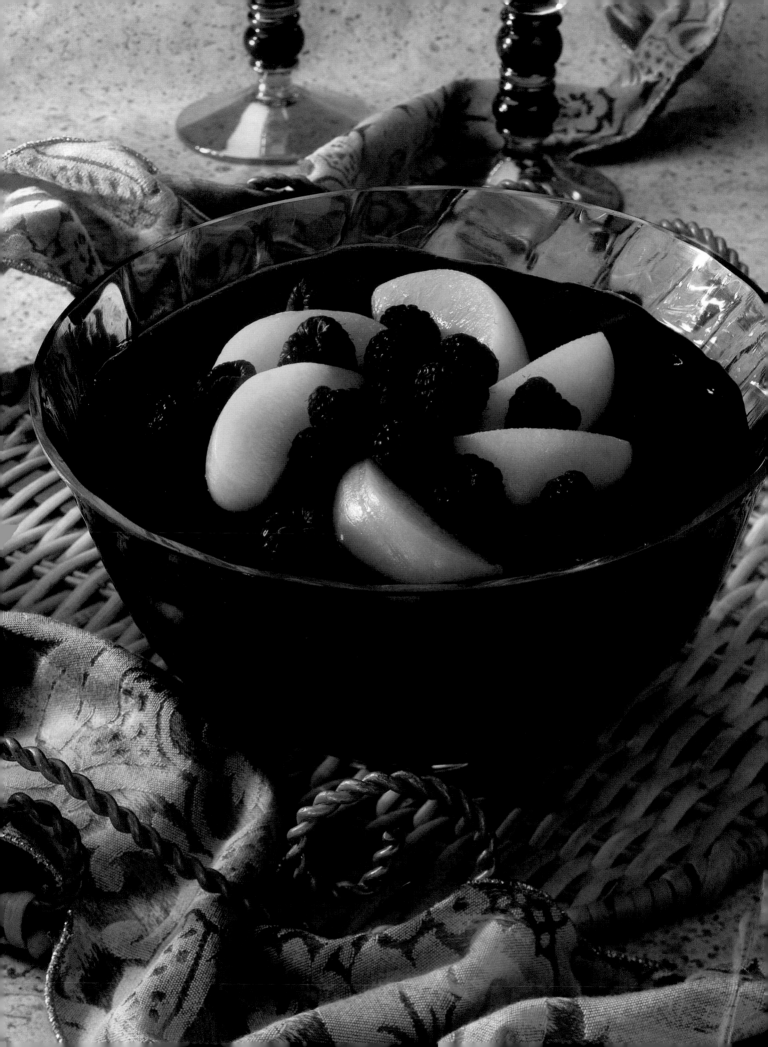

Pear-Ginger Upside-Down Cake

(Pictured on page 152)

2 unpeeled Bosc or Anjou pears, cored
and sliced 1/4-inch thick

3 tablespoons fresh lemon juice

1 to 2 tablespoons melted butter

1 to 2 tablespoons packed brown sugar

1 cup all-purpose flour

1 teaspoon baking powder

1 teaspoon ground cinnamon

1/4 teaspoon baking soda

1/8 teaspoon salt

1/3 cup fat-free milk

3 tablespoons no-sugar-added apricot
spread

1 egg

1 tablespoon vegetable oil

1 tablespoon minced fresh gingerroot or
3/4 teaspoon ground ginger

1. Preheat oven to 375°F. Spray 10-inch deep-dish pie pan with nonstick cooking spray.

2. Toss pears in lemon juice; drain. Brush butter evenly onto bottom of prepared pan; sprinkle sugar over butter. Arrange pears in pan; bake 10 minutes.

3. Meanwhile, combine flour, baking powder, cinnamon, baking soda and salt in small bowl; set aside. Combine milk, apricot spread, egg, oil and ginger in medium bowl; mix well. Add flour mixture; stir until well mixed (batter is very thick). Carefully spread batter evenly over pears to edge of pan.

4. Bake 20 to 25 minutes or until golden brown and toothpick inserted into center comes out clean.

5. Cool 5 minutes; use knife to loosen cake from side of pan. Place 10-inch plate over top of pan; quickly turn over to transfer cake to plate. Place any pears left in pan on top of cake. Serve warm. *Makes 8 servings*

Nutrients per Serving: 1 slice Cake (1/8 of total recipe)

Calories 139	**Fiber** 2g
Fat 4g (sat 1g)	**Cholesterol** 31mg
Protein 3g	**Sodium** 174mg
Carbohydrate 23g	

Exchanges: 1-1/2 starch, 1/2 fat

Oatmeal-Date Cookies

1/2 cup packed light brown sugar

1/4 cup margarine, softened

1 whole egg

1 egg white

1 tablespoon thawed frozen apple juice
concentrate

1 teaspoon vanilla extract

1-1/2 cups all-purpose flour

2 teaspoons baking soda

1/4 teaspoon salt

1-1/2 cups uncooked quick-cooking oats

1/2 cup chopped dates or raisins

1. Preheat oven to 350°F. Lightly coat cookie sheet with nonstick cooking spray; set aside.

2. Combine brown sugar and margarine in large bowl; mix well. Add egg, egg white, apple juice concentrate and vanilla; mix well.

3. Add flour, baking soda and salt; mix well. Stir in oats and dates. Drop dough by teaspoonfuls onto prepared cookie sheet.

4. Bake 8 to 10 minutes or until edges are very lightly browned. (Centers should still be soft.)

5. Cool 1 minute on cookie sheet. Remove to wire rack; cool completely.

Makes 3 dozen cookies

Nutrients per Serving: 1 Cookie

Calories 65	**Fiber** 1g
Fat 2g (sat <1g)	**Cholesterol** 6mg
Protein 1g	**Sodium** 106mg
Carbohydrate 11g	

Exchanges: 1 starch

Refrigerator Cookies

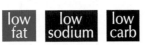

(Pictured at bottom right)

- 1/2 cup sugar
- 1/4 cup light corn syrup
- 1/4 cup margarine, softened
- 1/4 cup cholesterol-free egg substitute
- 1 teaspoon vanilla extract
- 1-3/4 cups all-purpose flour
- 1/4 teaspoon baking soda
- 1/4 teaspoon salt
- Cookie decorations (optional)

1. Beat sugar, corn syrup and margarine in large bowl. Add egg substitute and vanilla; mix well. Set aside.

2. Combine flour, baking soda and salt in medium bowl. Add to sugar mixture; mix well.

3. Form dough into 2 (1-1/2-inch-wide) rolls. Wrap in plastic wrap. Freeze 1 hour.

4. Preheat oven to 350°F. Line baking sheets with parchment paper. Cut dough into 1/4-inch-thick slices; place 1 inch apart on prepared cookie sheets. Sprinkle with cookie decorations, if desired.

5. Bake 8 to 10 minutes or until edges begin to turn golden brown. Cool on wire racks.

Makes about 4 dozen cookies

Variation: Add 2 tablespoons unsweetened cocoa powder to dough for chocolate cookies.

Nutrients per Serving: 1 Cookie (without decorations)

Calories 39	**Fiber** 0g
Fat 1g (sat 0g)	**Cholesterol** 0mg
Protein 0g	**Sodium** 32mg
Carbohydrate 7g	

Exchanges: 1/2 starch

White Chocolate Orange Mousse

Quick Recipe

- 1-1/2 cups cold fat-free milk
- 1 package (4-serving size) JELL-O® White Chocolate Flavor Fat Free Sugar Free Instant Reduced Calorie Pudding & Pie Filling
- 2 cups thawed COOL WHIP LITE® or COOL WHIP FREE® Whipped Topping
- 1 teaspoon grated orange peel

POUR milk into medium bowl. Add pudding mix. Beat with wire whisk 1 minute. Gently stir in whipped topping and orange peel. Spoon into 6 dessert dishes.

REFRIGERATE until ready to serve.

Makes 6 servings

Nutrients per Serving: 2/3 cup Mousse

Calories 90	**Fiber** 0g
Fat 3g (sat 3g)	**Cholesterol** 0mg
Protein 2g	**Sodium** 270mg
Carbohydrate 13g	

Exchanges: 1 starch, 1/2 fat

Refrigerator Cookies

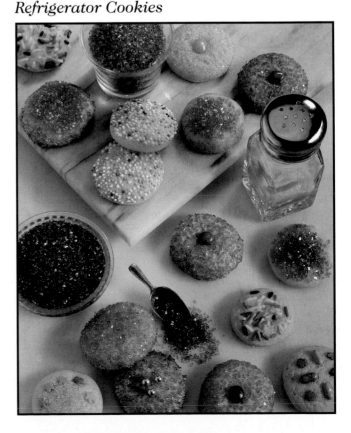

Luscious Chocolate Cheesecake

(Pictured at right)

2 cups (1 pound) nonfat cottage cheese

3/4 cup liquid egg substitute

2/3 cup sugar

4 ounces (1/2 of 8-ounce package) Neufchâtel cheese (1/3 less fat cream cheese), softened

1/3 cup HERSHEY'S Cocoa or HERSHEY'S Dutch Processed Cocoa

1/2 teaspoon vanilla extract

Yogurt Topping (recipe follows)

Sliced strawberries or mandarin orange segments (optional)

1. Heat oven to 300°F. Spray 9-inch springform pan with vegetable cooking spray.

2. Place cottage cheese, egg substitute, sugar, Neufchâtel cheese, cocoa and vanilla in food processor; process until smooth. Pour into prepared pan.

3. Bake 35 minutes or until edges are set.

4. Meanwhile, prepare Yogurt Topping. Carefully spread topping over cheesecake. Continue baking 5 minutes. Remove from oven to wire rack. With knife, loosen cheesecake from side of pan. Cool completely.

5. Cover; refrigerate until chilled. Remove side of pan. Serve with strawberries or mandarin orange segments, if desired. Refrigerate leftover cheesecake. *Makes 12 servings*

Yogurt Topping

2/3 cup plain fat-free yogurt

2 tablespoons sugar

1. Stir together yogurt and sugar in small bowl until well blended.

Nutrients per Serving: 1 slice Cheesecake (1/12 of total recipe) without strawberries or mandarin orange segments

Calories 84	**Fiber** <1g
Fat 2g (sat 1g)	**Cholesterol** 7mg
Protein 8g	**Sodium** 199mg
Carbohydrate 6g	

≈ ≈ ≈

Fruited Trifle

low sodium

1-3/4 cups fat-free milk

1 package (4-serving size) instant sugar-free vanilla pudding and pie filling

4 ounces reduced-fat cream cheese, softened

12 to 16 whole ladyfingers

2 cups fresh or frozen raspberries

1/2 cup thawed frozen fat-free nondairy whipped topping

1. Whisk together milk and pudding mix in large bowl. Beat in cream cheese with electric mixer at medium speed until smooth; set aside.

2. Place half the ladyfingers on bottom of 8- to 10-inch glass serving dish. Spread half the pudding mixture over ladyfingers. Arrange raspberries over pudding, reserving a few for garnish. Repeat layers with remaining ingredients.

3. Top with whipped topping. Refrigerate 1 hour. Garnish with reserved raspberries just before serving. *Makes 8 servings*

Nutrients per Serving: 1/8 of Trifle

Calories 145	**Fiber** 2g
Fat 4g (sat 2g)	**Cholesterol** 68mg
Protein 5g	**Sodium** 122mg
Carbohydrate 21g	

Exchanges: 1-1/2 starch, 1/2 fat

Luscious Chocolate Cheesecake

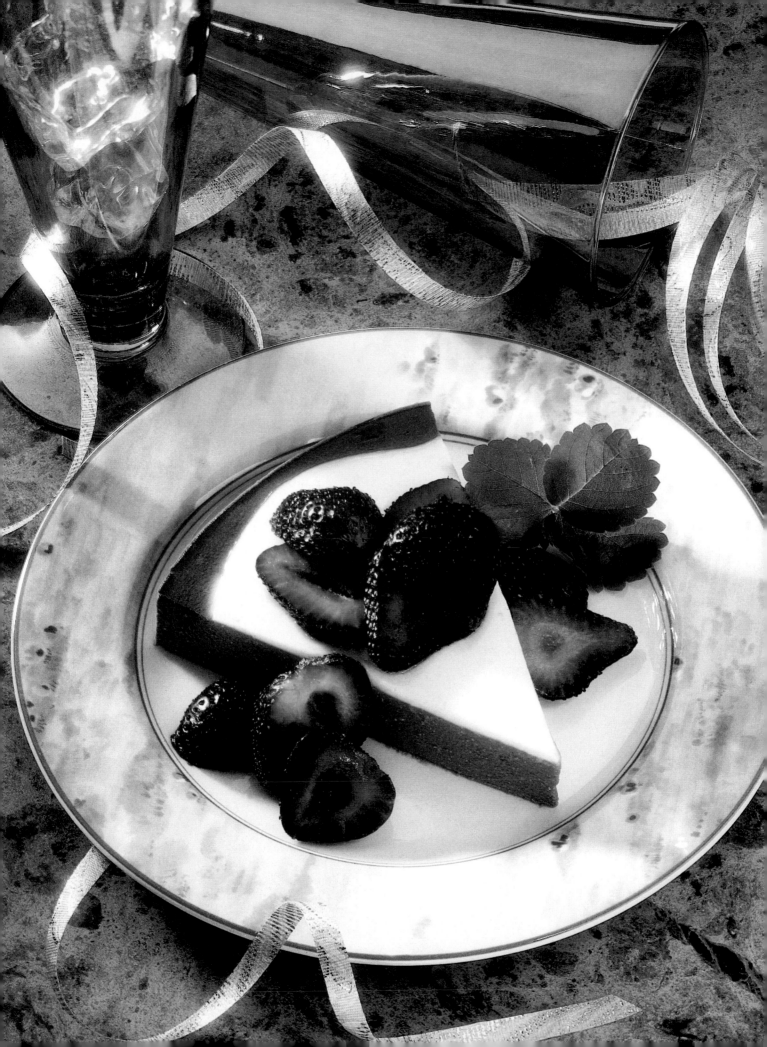

Tropical Fruit Coconut Tart

low sodium

(Pictured at right)

- **1 cup cornflakes, crushed**
- **1 can (3-1/2 ounces) sweetened flaked coconut**
- **2 egg whites**
- **1 can (15-1/4 ounces) pineapple tidbits in juice, undrained**
- **2 teaspoons cornstarch**
- **2 packets sugar substitute* *or* equivalent of 4 teaspoons sugar**
- **1 teaspoon coconut extract (optional)**
- **1 mango, peeled and thinly sliced**
- **1 medium banana, thinly sliced**
- **Pineapple leaves (optional)**

*This recipe was tested with Equal® sweetener.

1. Preheat oven to 425°F. Coat 9-inch springform pan with nonstick cooking spray; set aside.

2. Combine cereal, coconut and egg whites in medium bowl; toss gently to blend. Place coconut mixture in prepared pan; press firmly to coat bottom and 1/2 inch up side of pan.

3. Bake 8 minutes or until edge begins to brown. Cool completely on wire rack.

4. Drain pineapple, reserving pineapple juice. Combine pineapple juice and cornstarch in small saucepan; stir until cornstarch is dissolved. Bring to a boil over high heat. Continue boiling 1 minute, stirring constantly. Remove from heat; cool completely.

5. Stir in sugar substitute and coconut extract, if desired. Combine pineapple, mango slices and banana slices in medium bowl. Spoon into cooled crust; drizzle with pineapple sauce. Cover with plastic wrap and refrigerate 2 hours. Garnish with pineapple leaves, if desired.

Makes 8 servings

Note: The crust may be made 24 hours in advance, if desired.

Nutrients per Serving: 1 slice Tart (1/8 of total recipe)

Calories 139	**Fiber** 2g
Fat 4g (sat 3g)	**Cholesterol** 0mg
Protein 2g	**Sodium** 59mg
Carbohydrate 25g	

Exchanges: 1 starch, 1/2 fruit, 1 fat

Pumpkin Mousse Cups

low fat   low sodium

- **1 can (15 ounces) solid-pack pumpkin**
- **1/2 cup reduced-fat sweetened condensed milk**
- **4 packets sugar substitute* *or* equivalent of 8 teaspoons sugar**
- **1 teaspoon ground cinnamon**
- **1/4 teaspoon ground ginger**
- **1/4 teaspoon salt**
- **1 packet unflavored gelatin**
- **2 tablespoons water**
- **2 cups thawed frozen reduced-fat nondairy whipped topping**

*This recipe was tested with Equal® sweetener.

Microwave Directions
Combine pumpkin, milk, sugar substitute, cinnamon, ginger and salt in medium bowl; set aside. Combine gelatin and water in small microwavable bowl; let stand 2 minutes. Microwave at HIGH 40 seconds to dissolve gelatin. Stir into pumpkin mixture. Gently fold in whipped topping until well combined. Spoon into 8 small dessert dishes. Refrigerate 1 hour or until slightly firm.   *Makes 8 servings*

Note: This recipe was tested in an 1100-watt microwave oven.

Nutrients per Serving: 1 Mousse Cup (1/8 of total recipe)

Calories 113	**Fiber** 2g
Fat 2g (sat <1g)	**Cholesterol** 5mg
Protein 3g	**Sodium** 112mg
Carbohydrate 22g	

Exchanges: 1-1/2 starch

Tropical Fruit Coconut Tart

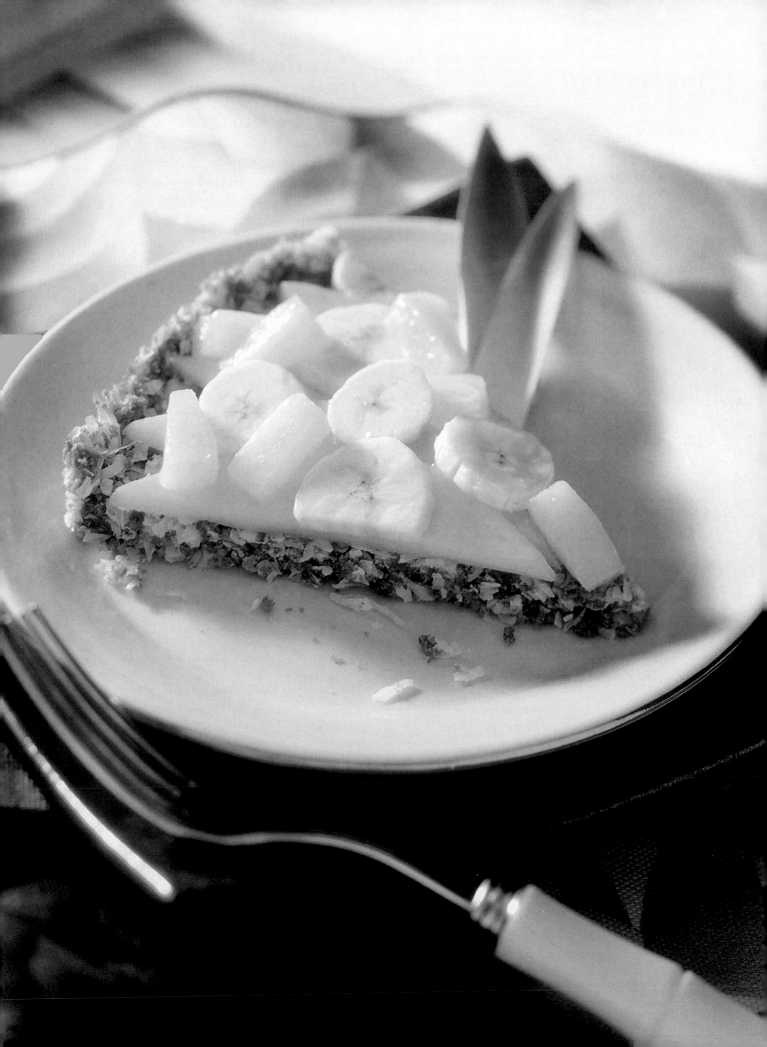

Yogurt Fluff

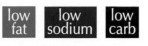

(Pictured at right)

3/4 cup boiling water
1 package (4-serving size) JELL-O® Brand Sugar Free Low Calorie Gelatin Dessert or JELL-O® Brand Gelatin Dessert, any flavor
1/2 cup cold water or fruit juice
  Ice cubes
1 container (8 ounces) BREYERS® Vanilla Lowfat Yogurt
1/2 teaspoon vanilla (optional)
5 tablespoons thawed COOL WHIP FREE® or COOL WHIP LITE® Whipped Topping

STIR boiling water into gelatin in large bowl at least 2 minutes until completely dissolved.

MIX cold water and ice cubes to make 1 cup.

ADD to gelatin, stirring until slightly thickened. Remove any remaining ice.

STIR in yogurt and vanilla. Pour into 5 dessert dishes.

REFRIGERATE 1-1/2 hours or until firm. Top with whipped topping.   *Makes 5 servings*

Nutrients per Serving: 1/2 cup Yogurt Fluff with 1 tablespoon Whipped Topping (made with JELL-O® Brand Sugar Free Low Calorie Gelatin Dessert, water and COOL WHIP FREE®)

Calories 61	**Fiber** 0g
Fat 1g (sat <1g)	**Cholesterol** 3mg
Protein 3g	**Sodium** 92mg
Carbohydrate 9g	

Exchanges: 1 starch

Cranberry Biscotti

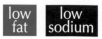

2-1/4 cups GOLD MEDAL® all-purpose flour
  3/4 cup sugar
    1 teaspoon baking powder
    1 teaspoon ground cinnamon
  1/2 teaspoon baking soda
    2 eggs
    2 egg whites
1-1/2 teaspoons almond extract
    1 cup FIBER ONE® cereal
  1/2 cup dried cranberries

1. Heat oven to 350°F. Spray cookie sheet with nonstick cooking spray.

2. Stir together flour, sugar, baking powder, cinnamon and baking soda in large bowl. Beat eggs, egg whites and almond extract with wire whisk until foamy. Stir egg mixture into flour mixture until well blended. Work in cereal and cranberries with hands. Place dough on floured surface. Knead lightly 8 to 10 times. Shape into one 16-inch roll or two 8-inch rolls. Place on cookie sheet. Flatten to about 1 inch thick.

3. Bake 30 minutes. Remove from cookie sheet; cool on wire rack 10 minutes. Cut into 1/2-inch slices. *Reduce oven temperature to 300°F.* Stand slices upright on cookie sheet; bake about 20 minutes longer or until crisp and light brown. Cool completely on wire rack.

Makes 32 cookies

Nutrients per Serving: 1 Cookie

Calories 67	**Fiber** 1g
Fat <1g (sat <1g)	**Cholesterol** 13mg
Protein 2g	**Sodium** 51mg
Carbohydrate 15g	

Exchanges: 1 starch

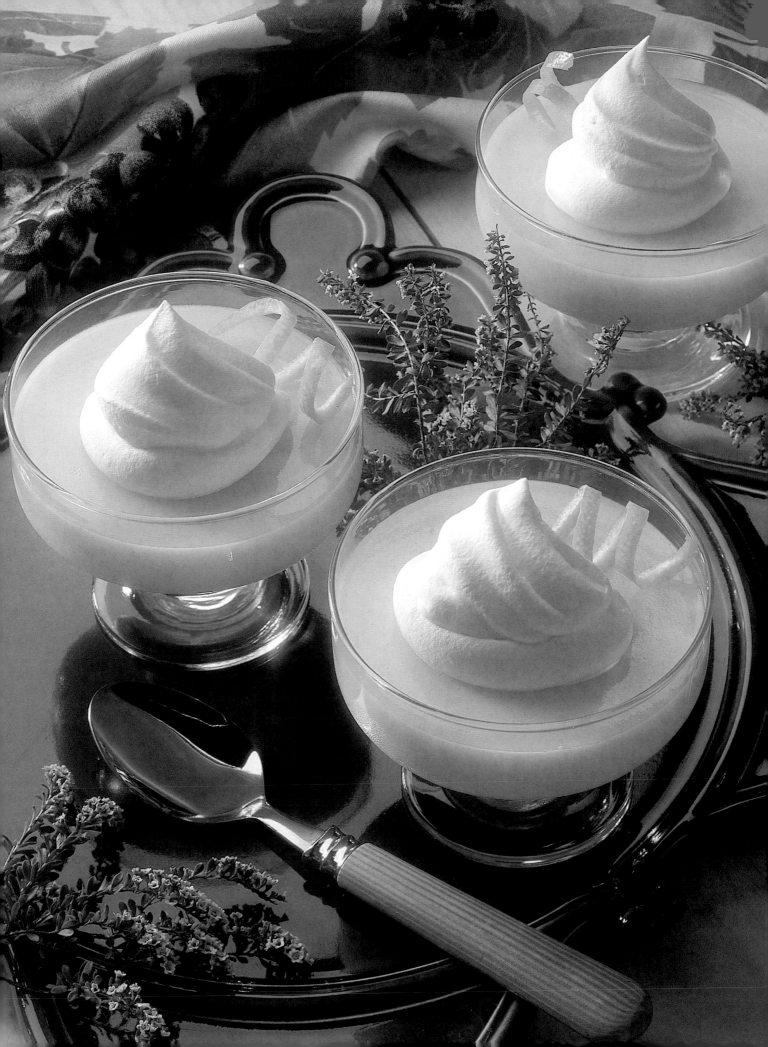

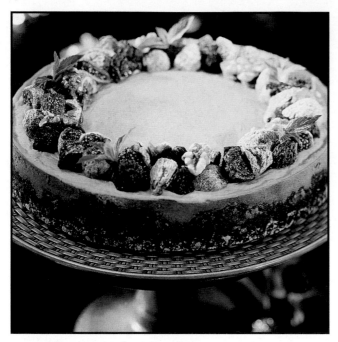

Pumpkin-Fig Cheesecake

Pumpkin-Fig Cheesecake

low fat

(Pictured above)

12 nonfat fig bar cookies

2 packages (8 ounces each) fat-free cream cheese, softened

1 package (8 ounces) reduced-fat cream cheese, softened

1 can (15 ounces) pumpkin

1 cup SPLENDA® No-Calorie Sweetener, granular form

1 cup cholesterol-free egg substitute

1/2 cup nonfat evaporated milk

1 tablespoon vanilla extract

2 teaspoons pumpkin pie spice mix

1/4 teaspoon salt

1/2 cup chopped dried figs

2 tablespoons walnut pieces

1. Preheat oven to 325°F. Lightly coat 8- to 9-inch springform baking pan with nonstick cooking spray.

2. Break up cookies with fingers, then chop by hand with knife or process in food processor until crumbly.

3. Lightly press crust onto bottom and side of pan. Bake 15 minutes; cool slightly while preparing filling.

4. In large bowl, beat cream cheese with mixer at high speed until smooth. Add pumpkin, SPLENDA®, egg substitute, milk, vanilla, spice mix and salt. Beat until smooth. Spread filling evenly over crust.

5. Place springform pan on baking sheet. Bake 1 hour and 15 minutes or until top begins to crack and center moves very little when pan is jiggled.

6. Cool on wire rack to room temperature; refrigerate 4 to 6 hours or overnight before serving.

7. Just before serving, sprinkle top with figs and nuts. *Makes 16 slices*

Nutrients per Serving: 1 slice Cheesecake (1/16 of total recipe)

Calories 157	**Fiber** 2g
Fat 3g (sat 2g)	**Cholesterol** 9mg
Protein 9g	**Sodium** 310mg
Carbohydrate 22g	

Exchanges: 1-1/2 starch, 1 lean meat

Tip

Splenda® Granular, the no-calorie sweetener used in this recipe, is one brand of sucralose on the market today. Sucralose is touted for its superior baking qualities and can be substituted measure-for-measure for regular granulated sugar.

Cool 'n' Easy® Strawberry Pie

2/3 cup boiling water
1 package (4-serving size) JELL-O® Brand Strawberry Flavor Sugar Free Low Calorie Gelatin
1/2 cup cold water
  Ice cubes
1 tub (8 ounces) COOL WHIP LITE® Whipped Topping, thawed, divided
1 cup chopped strawberries
1 prepared reduced-fat graham cracker crumb crust (6 ounce or 9 inch)
5 whole strawberries, halved

STIR boiling water into gelatin in large bowl at least 2 minutes until completely dissolved. Mix cold water and ice to make 1 cup. Add to gelatin, stirring until slightly thickened. Remove any remaining ice.

STIR in 2-1/2 cups of the whipped topping with wire whisk until smooth. Mix in chopped strawberries. Refrigerate 15 to 20 minutes or until mixture is very thick and will mound. Spoon into crust.

REFRIGERATE 4 hours or overnight. Garnish with remaining whipped topping and strawberry halves. Store leftover pie in refrigerator.

Makes 8 servings

Nutrients per Serving: 1 slice Pie (1/8 of total recipe)

Calories 130	**Fiber** 1g
Fat 5g (sat 2g)	**Cholesterol** 0mg
Protein 2g	**Sodium** 130mg
Carbohydrate 21g	

Exchanges: 1-1/2 starch, 1/2 fat

French Vanilla Freeze

10-3/4 teaspoons EQUAL® FOR RECIPES *or* 36 packets EQUAL® sweetener *or* 1-1/2 cups EQUAL® SPOONFUL™
2 tablespoons cornstarch
1 piece vanilla bean (2 inches)
1/8 teaspoon salt
2 cups skim milk
2 tablespoons margarine
1 cup real liquid egg product
1 teaspoon vanilla

• Combine Equal®, cornstarch, vanilla bean and salt in medium saucepan; stir in milk and margarine. Heat to boiling over medium-high heat, whisking constantly. Boil until thickened, whisking constantly, about 1 minute.

• Whisk about 1 cup milk mixture into egg product in small bowl; whisk egg mixture back into milk mixture in saucepan. Cook over very low heat, whisking constantly, 30 to 60 seconds or until mixture reaches 160°F. Remove from heat and stir in vanilla. Let cool; remove vanilla bean. Refrigerate until chilled, about 1 hour.

• Freeze mixture in ice cream maker according to manufacturer's directions. Pack into freezer container and freeze until firm, 8 hours or overnight. Before serving, let stand at room temperature until slightly softened, about 15 minutes. *Makes 6 (1/2-cup) servings*

Nutrients per Serving: 1/2 cup Freeze

Calories 123	**Fiber** <1g
Fat 4g (sat 1g)	**Cholesterol** 1mg
Protein 12g	**Sodium** 203mg
Carbohydrate 4g	

Exchanges: 1/2 milk, 1 lean meat

JELL-O® 'n Juice Parfaits

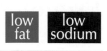

(Pictured at right)

2 cups boiling water, divided
1 package (4-serving size) JELL-O® Brand Strawberry Flavor Sugar Free Low Calorie Gelatin
1 package (4-serving size) JELL-O® Brand Lemon Flavor Sugar Free Low Calorie Gelatin
2 cups cold apple juice, divided
1 tub (8 ounces) COOL WHIP FREE® Whipped Topping, thawed

STIR 1 cup boiling water into each of the strawberry and lemon gelatins in separate bowls at least 2 minutes until completely dissolved. Stir 1 cup apple juice into each bowl. Pour into separate 9-inch square pans.

REFRIGERATE 4 hours or until firm. Cut gelatin in each pan into 1/2-inch cubes. Layer alternating flavors of gelatin and whipped topping in 8 dessert glasses. Garnish with additional whipped topping, if desired.

Makes 8 servings

Nutrients per Serving: 1 Parfait

Calories 85	**Fiber** <1g
Fat <1g (sat <1g)	**Cholesterol** 0mg
Protein 1g	**Sodium** 67mg
Carbohydrate 17g	

Exchanges: 1 starch

Tip

"Parfait" is the French word for "perfect." Layered in tall, footed, clear glasses known as parfait glasses, the traditional French version of this dish is made with egg yolks, sugar, whipped cream and flavoring. JELL-O® 'n Juice Parfaits are a fresh and light twist on this classic.

Mocha Crinkles

1-1/3 cups packed light brown sugar
1/2 cup canola oil
1/4 cup reduced-fat sour cream
1 egg
1 teaspoon vanilla extract
1-3/4 cups all-purpose flour
3/4 cup unsweetened cocoa powder
2 teaspoons instant espresso or coffee granules
1 teaspoon baking soda
1/4 teaspoon salt
1/8 teaspoon black pepper
1/2 cup powdered sugar

1. Beat brown sugar and oil in medium bowl with electric mixer. Mix in sour cream, egg and vanilla. Set aside.

2. Mix flour, cocoa, espresso, baking soda, salt and pepper in another medium bowl.

3. Add flour mixture to brown sugar mixture; mix well. Refrigerate dough until firm, 3 to 4 hours.

4. Preheat oven to 350°F. Pour powdered sugar into shallow bowl. Set aside. Roll dough into 1-inch balls. Roll balls in powdered sugar.

5. Bake on ungreased cookie sheets 10 to 12 minutes or until tops of cookies are firm to touch. (Do not overbake.) Cool on wire racks.

Makes about 6 dozen cookies

Nutrients per Serving: 1 Cookie

Calories 44	**Fiber** 0g
Fat 1g (sat <1g)	**Cholesterol** 3mg
Protein 0g	**Sodium** 28mg
Carbohydrate 7g	

Exchanges: 1/2 starch

JELL-O® 'n Juice Parfait

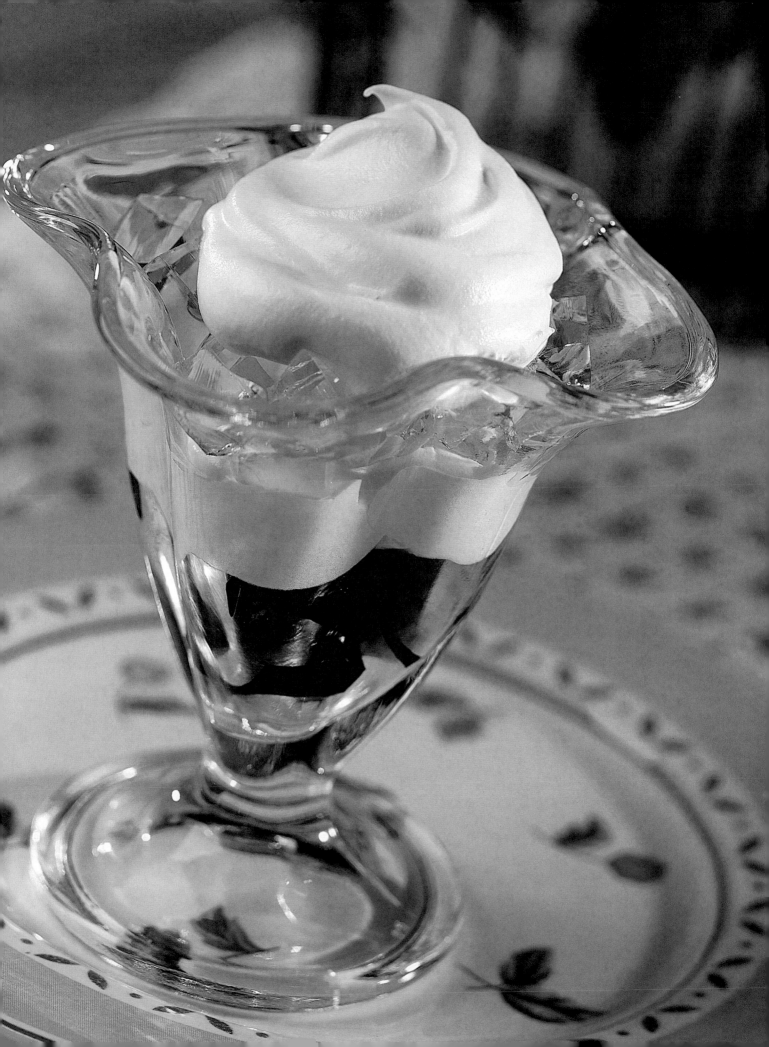

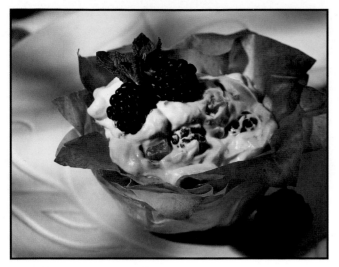

Blackberry Strudel Cup

Blackberry Strudel Cups

(Pictured above)

6 sheets frozen phyllo dough, thawed
   Nonstick cooking spray
1 pint blackberries
2 tablespoons sugar
1 cup thawed frozen reduced-fat
   nondairy whipped topping
1 container (6 ounces) custard-style
   apricot- or peach-flavored
   reduced-fat yogurt
   Mint sprigs for garnish

1. Preheat oven to 400°F. Cut phyllo dough crosswise into 4 pieces. Place 1 sheet phyllo dough on work surface. Keep remaining sheets covered with plastic wrap and damp kitchen towel. Lightly coat first sheet with cooking spray; place in large custard cup. Place second sheet on top of first, alternating corners; spray with cooking spray. Repeat with remaining 2 phyllo sheets, continuing to alternate corners. Repeat with remaining phyllo dough to form 6 strudel cups. Place custard cups on cookie sheet; bake about 15 minutes or until pastry is golden. Let cool to room temperature.

2. Meanwhile, combine blackberries and sugar in small bowl; let stand 15 minutes. Mix whipped topping and yogurt in medium bowl. Reserve 1/2 cup blackberries for garnish; gently

stir remaining blackberries into whipped topping mixture. Spoon into cooled pastry cups. Garnish with reserved blackberries and mint sprigs. *Makes 6 servings*

Nutrients per Serving: 1 Strudel Cup

Calories 125	**Fiber** 3g
Fat 4g (sat <1g)	**Cholesterol** 3mg
Protein 3g	**Sodium** 22mg
Carbohydrate 25g	

Exchanges: 1-1/2 fruit, 1 fat

Butterscotch Crispies

2 cups sifted all-purpose flour
1 teaspoon baking soda
1 teaspoon salt
1/2 cup margarine, softened
2-1/2 cups packed light brown sugar
2 eggs
1 teaspoon vanilla extract
2 cups quick-cooking rolled oats
2 cups puffed rice cereal
1/2 cup chopped walnuts

Preheat oven to 350°F. Sift flour, baking soda and salt onto waxed paper. Cream margarine and brown sugar with electric mixer at medium speed in large bowl until fluffy. Beat in eggs, 1 at a time, until fluffy. Stir in vanilla.

Add flour mixture, 1/3 at a time, until well blended; stir in rolled oats, rice cereal and walnuts. Drop by teaspoonfuls, about 1 inch apart, onto large cookie sheets lightly sprayed with nonstick cooking spray. Bake 10 minutes or until cookies are firm and lightly golden. Remove to wire racks; cool.

Makes 8-1/2 dozen cookies

Favorite recipe from **The Sugar Association, Inc.**

Nutrients per Serving: 1 Cookie

Calories 50	**Fiber** <1g
Fat 1g (sat <1g)	**Cholesterol** 4mg
Protein 1g	**Sodium** 49mg
Carbohydrate 9g	

Exchanges: 1/2 starch, 1/2 fat

Acknowledgments

*The publisher would like to thank the companies and organizations
listed below for the use of their recipes and photographs
in this publication.*

Butterball® Turkey Company

Colorado Potato Administrative Committee

ConAgra Foods®

Del Monte Corporation

Egg Beaters®

Equal® sweetener

Fleischmann's® Yeast

General Mills, Inc.

Guiltless Gourmet®

Hershey Foods Corporation

Kraft Foods Holdings

McIlhenny Company (TABASCO® brand Pepper Sauce)

Minnesota Cultivated Wild Rice Council

Mushroom Council

National Pork Board

NatraTaste® is a registered trademark of Stadt Corporation

North Dakota Wheat Commission

The Quaker® Oatmeal Kitchens

The J.M. Smucker Company

Splenda® is a registered trademark of McNeil Nutritionals

The Sugar Association, Inc.

Uncle Ben's Inc.

USA Rice Federation

Wisconsin Milk Marketing Board

General Index

Index **185**

186 *Index*

Alphabetical Index

METRIC CONVERSION CHART

VOLUME MEASUREMENTS (dry)

1/8 teaspoon = 0.5 mL
1/4 teaspoon = 1 mL
1/2 teaspoon = 2 mL
3/4 teaspoon = 4 mL
1 teaspoon = 5 mL
1 tablespoon = 15 mL
2 tablespoons = 30 mL
1/4 cup = 60 mL
1/3 cup = 75 mL
1/2 cup = 125 mL
2/3 cup = 150 mL
3/4 cup = 175 mL
1 cup = 250 mL
2 cups = 1 pint = 500 mL
3 cups = 750 mL
4 cups = 1 quart = 1 L

VOLUME MEASUREMENTS (fluid)

1 fluid ounce (2 tablespoons) = 30 mL
4 fluid ounces (1/2 cup) = 125 mL
8 fluid ounces (1 cup) = 250 mL
12 fluid ounces (1 1/2 cups) = 375 mL
16 fluid ounces (2 cups) = 500 mL

WEIGHTS (mass)

1/2 ounce = 15 g
1 ounce = 30 g
3 ounces = 90 g
4 ounces = 120 g
8 ounces = 225 g
10 ounces = 285 g
12 ounces = 360 g
16 ounces = 1 pound = 450 g

DIMENSIONS

1/16 inch = 2 mm
1/8 inch = 3 mm
1/4 inch = 6 mm
1/2 inch = 1.5 cm
3/4 inch = 2 cm
1 inch = 2.5 cm

OVEN TEMPERATURES

250°F = 120°C
275°F = 140°C
300°F = 150°C
325°F = 160°C
350°F = 180°C
375°F = 190°C
400°F = 200°C
425°F = 220°C
450°F = 230°C

BAKING PAN SIZES

Utensil	Size in Inches/Quarts	Metric Volume	Size in Centimeters
Baking or Cake Pan (square or rectangular)	8 × 8 × 2	2 L	20 × 20 × 5
	9 × 9 × 2	2.5 L	23 × 23 × 5
	12 × 8 × 2	3 L	30 × 20 × 5
	13 × 9 × 2	3.5 L	33 × 23 × 5
Loaf Pan	8 × 4 × 3	1.5 L	20 × 10 × 7
	9 × 5 × 3	2 L	23 × 13 × 7
Round Layer Cake Pan	8 × 1 1/2	1.2 L	20 × 4
	9 × 1 1/2	1.5 L	23 × 4
Pie Plate	8 × 1 1/4	750 mL	20 × 3
	9 × 1 1/4	1 L	23 × 3
Baking Dish or Casserole	1 quart	1 L	—
	1 1/2 quart	1.5 L	—
	2 quart	2 L	—